STANDARDS OF ACCOUNTING AND FINANCIAL REPORTING for VOLUNTARY HEALTH AND WELFARE ORGANIZATIONS

Revised 1988
Third Edition

STANDARDS OF ACCOUNTING AND FINANCIAL REPORTING for VOLUNTARY HEALTH AND WELFARE ORGANIZATIONS

Revised 1988—Third Edition

National Health Council, Inc.
National Assembly of National Voluntary Health and Social Welfare Organizations, Inc.
United Way of America

Published by the National Health Council, Inc.,
622 Third Avenue, New York, NY 10017

Manufactured in the United States of America

Library of Congress Cataloging in Publication Data
Standards of accounting and financial reporting for
voluntary health and welfare organizations.
1. Voluntary health agencies—Accounting—Standards—United States. 2. Charities—Accounting—Standards—United States. I. National Health Council (U.S.)
HF5686.C3S7 1988 657'.832 88-13572

ISBN 0-929852-00-1

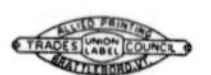

Foreword

The movement to establish uniform standards of accounting and financial reporting for voluntary nonprofit organizations spans over a quarter of a century. The publication of *Standards* in 1964 was a landmark event. Prior to that, these organizations had no formal guidance with respect to accounting and financial reporting. Practice varied widely at the sub-sector level of the "industry" and varied even within the sub-sectors. Since the publication of *Standards* in 1964, a measure of uniformity and consistency in reporting has developed among voluntary health and welfare organizations.

Over the years, interest in public accountability for funds used for philanthropic purposes has also increased. At the same time, *Standards* gained wide acceptance not only among affected agencies but among various funders of voluntary charities, monitoring bodies and state charity regulators.

In 1974, the American Institute of Certified Public Accountants (AICPA) published the revised industry audit guide called "Audits of Voluntary Health and Welfare Organizations." This guide described and effectively established the *generally accepted accounting principles (GAAP)* applicable to financial reporting by health and welfare organizations. The audit guide observed that, in most instances, these principles (GAAP) were compatible with those set forth in *Standards* and that the authors of *Standards* had advised the AICPA Committee that it was their intent to revise *Standards*, as necessary, to achieve maximum uniformity with that guide. In keeping with this commitment, *Standards* was revised in 1974 to achieve compatibility with the 1974 AICPA guide.

Over the years, since the publication of the Revised 1974 *Standards,* a number of significant developments have taken place, among them:

1. The Financial Accounting Standards Board (FASB) was created as the standard-setting body for accounting and financial reporting. FASB has launched a number of initiatives in the nonprofit accounting arena.

2. In 1981, the AICPA issued *Audits of Certain Nonprofit Organizations.*
3. A number of issues have arisen which deal with reporting practices and need clarification. In particular, prior guidance pertaining to the accounting for "joint costs" resulted in divergent practices. This matter has now been resolved with the formulation of Statement of Position (SOP) 87-2, "Accounting for Joint Costs of Informational Materials and Activities of Not-for-Profit Organizations that Include a Fund-Raising Appeal," issued by the AICPA in August 1987 after years of deliberations.

The Revised 1974 *Standards,* in its "Foreword," observed that over time "it can be expected that further changes may be made in *Standards* as experience and adjudication produce new practices and rules." The events and experience of the past fourteen years indicated that it was time to take a fresh look at *Standards* and to publish a third edition, reflecting current authoritative literature for accounting and financial reporting by voluntary health and welfare agencies.

Thus, in the Fall of 1985, the three sponsors launched a project to revise and publish the third edition of *Standards.* United Way of America agreed to serve as project secretariat and assigned a senior staff member, Russy D. Sumariwalla, as the project director. A top-ranking Joint Liaison Committee was selected, composed of ten experts chosen from among executive finance managers of major agencies and public accountants well-versed in the specialty of nonprofit accounting.

The Joint Liaison Committee was given complete freedom to review all relevant literature and to develop a manuscript that incorporates the most recent thinking on the subject. The Committee spent countless hours over a three-year period developing and refining the manuscript. Earlier drafts of the manuscript were shared with relevant groups including representatives of the affected organizations and regulatory and standard-setting bodies. Many excellent suggestions were received and incorporated into the final document.

The three sponsors are deeply indebted to the members of the Joint Liaison Committee for their dedicated efforts in producing a document which will make an important contribution to the voluntary health and welfare sector. We are also thankful to the many individuals who took time to offer useful comments on drafts.

Finally, the sponsors want to express their appreciation to Russy D. Sumariwalla, whose expert guidance through a complex process helped to bring this product to fruition. His knowledge of the voluntary health and welfare field, his clear grasp of the substantive issues, and his management skills were enormously useful to the deliberations of the Joint Liaison Committee and the sponsors.

With the publication of this third edition, we reaffirm our commitment to the highest standards of public accountability for funds used by the voluntary health and welfare sector.

JOHN R. GARRISON
President
National Health Council, Inc.

SOLON B. COUSINS
President
National Assembly of National Voluntary Health and Social Welfare Organizations, Inc.

EDWARD A. BRENNAN
Chairman of the Board of Governors
United Way of America

September 1988

STANDARDS OF ACCOUNTING AND FINANCIAL REPORTING FOR VOLUNTARY HEALTH AND WELFARE ORGANIZATIONS

Revised 1988 Third Edition

JOINT LIAISON COMMITTEE

MATTHEW G. MCCROSSON, CHAIR
Treasurer and Secretary
March of Dimes Birth Defects Foundation
White Plains, New York

GUY A. BENSON
Senior Vice President—Finance
United Way of Tri-State, Inc.
New York, New York

IRWIN BROD
Senior Vice President
Brakeley, John Price Jones Inc.
Stamford, Connecticut

JOHN D. CAMPBELL
Director, Accounting Division
American Red Cross
Alexandria, Virginia

HERBERT K. FOLPE
Partner
Peat Marwick Main & Co.
New York, New York

ANNE FARLEY
Senior Manager
Peat Marwick Main & Co.
New York, New York

LIEUTENANT COLONEL EDWARD J. JOHNSON
Secretary for Business Administration
Salvation Army U.S.A.—Southern Territory
Atlanta, Georgia

RICHARD F. LARKIN
Senior Manager
Nonprofit Industry Services Group
Price Waterhouse
Bethesda, Maryland

GARY D. MALLERY
Partner
Deloitte, Haskins & Sells
Baltimore, Maryland

TIMOTHY J. RACEK
Partner
Arthur Andersen & Co.
New York, New York

Project Secretariat—RUSSY D. SUMARIWALLA, STAFF DIRECTOR
Standards Revision Project, United Way Institute, United Way of America, Alexandria, Virginia

CONTENTS

Chapter IV
THE CLASSIFICATION AND REPORTING OF PUBLIC SUPPORT AND OTHER REVENUE

Chapter V

CHAPTER I

THE PURPOSE OF THE REVISED STANDARDS

This third edition of *Standards of Accounting and Financial Reporting for Voluntary Health and Welfare Organizations* (*Standards*) was prepared to continue the mission of the previous editions—to attain uniform accounting and external financial reporting in compliance with generally accepted accounting principles by all voluntary health and welfare organizations. The intended constituencies of *Standards*, as indicated by its title, are voluntary health and welfare organizations, including those organizations which are members of or are affiliated with the National Health Council, Inc., the National Assembly of National Voluntary Health and Social Welfare Organizations, Inc., and the United Way of America. Since 1964, *Standards* has guided these organizations' financial reporting. *Standards* has been successful in achieving uniformity and comparability of financial reporting within the industry and, with it, increased public understanding of and confidence in the organizations' financial reports. The third edition was necessitated by new and emerging accounting issues that have evolved over the 14 years since the second edition was published.

DEVELOPMENT OF STANDARDS

Standards, first published in 1964, was the original comprehensive compilation of accounting principles and financial reporting practices for voluntary health and welfare agencies. In 1967, the American Institute of Certified Public Accountants (AICPA) published the audit guide, *Audits of Voluntary Health and Welfare Organizations*, for the industry; this guide neither endorsed nor disagreed with *Standards* but stated:

> The prescribed standard accounting and reporting practices will, if consistently applied, result in reducing the variety of reporting practices since *Standards* provides, in general, only one method of application of certain practices.

With the publication of a revision of the AICPA audit guide in 1974, the question of varying principles appeared to be largely resolved, as indicated by the following excerpt from the audit guide:

> The revised audit guide describes generally accepted accounting principles applicable to financial reporting of health and welfare organizations. In most instances, these principles are compatible with those set forth in the *Standards of Accounting and Financial Reporting for Voluntary Health and Welfare Organizations*. The National Health Council and the National Assembly have advised that it is their intent to revise the *Standards*, as necessary, to achieve the maximum possible uniformity with this guide.

As promised, the sponsors shortly thereafter revised *Standards* with the intent of conforming it to the 1974 revised audit guide.

NEED FOR CURRENT REVISION

Since the revision of *Standards* in 1974, certain inconsistencies have developed in practice between *Standards* and the 1974 audit guide. Many organizations came to view the audit guide as providing different treatment in certain areas, primarily allocation of joint costs of multi-purpose informational activities. In addition, since 1974, the Financial Accounting Standards Board (FASB) and the AICPA have made significant additions to the authoritative accounting literature that affect all not-for-profit organizations.

The FASB, formed in 1973 to function as the accounting standards setting body, has issued over ninety Statements of Financial Accounting Standards (SFAS), many of which are relevant to voluntary health and welfare agencies. Several of the statements, including No. 13 on leases, No. 43 on compensated absences, No. 74 on special termination benefits, and No. 87 on pension plans, addressed transactions entered into by voluntary health and welfare organizations that are not specifically covered in *Standards*. FASB Statement No. 32 gave additional authoritative status to the AICPA's audit guide by declaring the accounting principles set forth in the audit guide as preferable when justifying changes in accounting principles.

Perhaps more important to the industry in the long run are the FASB Financial Accounting Concepts projects that do not result in immediate standards, but provide a conceptual framework on which future uniform accounting principles for all not-for-profit organizations will be based. FASB Statement of Financial Accounting Concepts No. 4, "Objectives of Financial Reporting by Nonbusiness Organizations," issued in December 1980, was the first concepts statement to specifically address financial statements of not-for-profit organizations. Concepts Statement No. 4, which focused on the needs of users, concluded that general purpose financial reporting by not-for-profit organizations should provide information to resource providers and others that is useful in:

- Making decisions about allocating resources to these organizations.
- Assessing the services these organizations provide and their ability to continue to provide those services (financial viability).
- Assessing how managers of these organizations discharge their stewardship responsibilities.

Concepts Statement No. 4 also concluded that the information needed to achieve those objectives include an explanation of:

- Economic resources, obligations, and net resources of an organization and the effects of transactions, events, and circumstances that change resources and interests in those resources.
- The performance of an organization during a period. Periodic measurement of the changes in the amount and nature of the net resources of a nonbusiness organization and information about the service efforts and accomplishments of an organization *together* [emphasis added] represent the information most useful in assessing performance.
- How an organization obtains and spends cash or other liquid resources, its borrowing and repayment of borrowing, and other factors that may affect an organization's liquidity.

When applied specifically to voluntary health and welfare agencies, Concepts Statement No. 4 supports and refines long-standing views about the appropriate objectives of financial reporting for these agencies, the best vehicles for communicating the information, and the audience of financial statement users.

Users of agencies' financial statements include contributors, federated fund-raising organizations, other donor groups, organizations affiliated with the agency, contributor information bodies, state and other governmental charities regulators, beneficiaries, lenders and suppliers. Federal and state grant-making agencies also have become an important category of user. And finally, as indicated in Concepts Statement No. 4, governing boards may also be important users of general purpose financial reports as they carry out their fiduciary responsibilities.

In addition, in 1985, the FASB issued its Concepts Statement No. 6 "Elements of Financial Statements," which defines ten elements of financial statements, seven of which are applicable to not-for-profit organizations—assets, liabilities, net assets, revenues, expenses, gains and losses—and classifies net assets into three classes: unrestricted, temporarily restricted, permanently restricted. The FASB, with the assistance of the AICPA, will use the concepts in this Statement as the basis for a set of uniform accounting and financial reporting principles applicable to all not-for-profit organizations. Ultimately, consistency in financial reporting within the voluntary health and welfare industry will give way to consistency in financial reporting among all not-for-profit organizations. Additional revisions to *Standards* will be needed as FASB standards evolve.

Also since the second edition of *Standards*, the AICPA has published another audit guide, *Audits of Certain Nonprofit Organizations*, and a companion Statement of Position No. 78-10, *Accounting Principles and Reporting Practices for Certain Nonprofit Organizations*, applicable to those nonprofit organizations not covered by the college and university, hospital, state and local government, or voluntary health and welfare audit guides. Publication of this document has created uncertainty over which organizations are covered by *Standards* and *Audits of Voluntary Health and Welfare Organizations*, a matter which is further addressed later in this chapter.

Finally, in 1981, since the second edition, the IRS and most states agreed to accept IRS Form 990, *Return of Organization Exempt from Income Tax*, as a uniform annual report. Many state regulators revised their annual reports to use Form 990 as the basic reporting document. Some states devised additional schedules that were to be completed, and many required the organization's auditor to opine on Form 990. The Internal Revenue Service adopted essentially the voluntary health and welfare audit guide reporting model for Form 990.

AUTHORITATIVE STATUS, MATERIALITY AND APPLICABILITY

This edition also clarifies two areas of confusion—the authoritative status of *Standards* and the organizations to which it is applicable. With regard to authoritative status, *Standards* does not establish "Generally Accepted Accounting Principles"—currently the function of the Financial Accounting Standards Board (FASB)—but rather, provides additional explanation of current authoritative literature and illustrations particularly applicable to voluntary health and welfare organizations. *Standards* focuses on general purpose financial statements; it does not include guidance for management reporting, budgeting, or data processing.

Materiality

Generally accepted accounting principles typically apply to transactions or balances which are material to the entity in question, i.e., knowledge of which would influence the judgment of an informed user of the financial statements. Similarly, the guidance and explanations in *Standards* are intended to apply to material items. In evaluating the materiality of departures from *Standards*, both quantitative and qualitative factors should be considered, such as the dollar effects, the significance of the item, the pervasiveness of the departure, and the impact of the departure taken as a whole. However, because voluntary health and welfare organizations are not profit oriented, quantitative benchmarks are normally determined from bases other than excess of revenue over expenses. Other appropriate benchmarks might include total revenue, expenses, assets, or fund balances for a particular fund, or for all funds combined.

Applicability

Organizations to which *Standards* is applicable are essentially the same voluntary health and welfare organizations that follow the AICPA audit guide, *Audits of Voluntary Health and Welfare Organizations*. The voluntary health and welfare audit guide defines its scope as follows:

> ". . . organizations formed for the purpose of performing voluntary services for various segments of society. They are tax-exempt (organized for the benefit of the public), supported by the public, and operated on a 'not-for-profit' basis. Most voluntary health and welfare organizations concentrate their efforts and expend their resources in an attempt to solve health and welfare problems of our society and, in many cases, those of specific individuals. As a group, voluntary health and welfare organizations include those nonprofit organizations that derive their revenue primarily from voluntary contributions from the general public to be used for general or specific purposes connected with health, welfare, or community services."

Difficulties in determining whether an organization meets the audit guide "definition" arise because the operative phrases, "primarily from voluntary contributions from the general public" and "health, welfare or community services," are not precisely defined.

To assist in identifying those organizations that should follow the voluntary health and welfare audit guide and *Standards*, this edition offers the following additional guidance:

- Agencies that are members of or affiliated with the National Health Council, Inc., the National Assembly of National Voluntary Health and Social Welfare Organizations, Inc., and the United Way of America, should follow the provisions of *Standards*, unless they are clearly covered by another AICPA audit guide or statement of position.
- Organizations should evaluate whether a substantial amount of their revenue is normally from voluntary contributions from the general public and whether a significant part of their organization's mission includes the rendering of health, welfare, or community services.
- Voluntary contributions from the general public include direct public gifts as well as allocations or transfers. The latter is a sharing of contributions from the general public with the organization from fund-raising or affiliated organizations. In most cases, amounts reported as public support on the organization's Statement of Revenue and Expenses and Changes in Fund

Balances would qualify as voluntary contributions. In determining whether these *Standards* are applicable to the organization, amounts received from private foundations, corporations, or board members are normally considered voluntary contributions from the general public.

- Community services excludes those services specifically addressed in AICPA Statement of Position 78-10—museums, research organizations, etc.—as well as those referenced or implied in the hospital audit guide and colleges and universities audit guide.

An organization should use this guidance, along with facts relevant to its own situation, when determining whether it should be classified as a voluntary health and welfare organization. Its determination should then be followed consistently unless there are significant changes in its sources of support or in the types of its program services.

It is recognized that a number of organizations which otherwise are viewed as voluntary health and welfare organizations may not receive a substantial amount of their revenues from contributions from the general public, due to receipt of significant fees from clients, governmental support or other revenue. Unless these agencies are among the organizations which are specifically listed as covered by another AICPA audit guide, the use of these *Standards* to govern their financial reporting is preferable until such time as FASB completes its projects to establish uniform accounting principles for all nonprofit organizations.

SUMMARY OF SIGNIFICANT CHANGES AND CLARIFICATIONS

All of these developments and the issues raised since the first revision in 1974 point up the need to again revise *Standards*. In revising *Standards* to address the events of the past decade, the essential framework of the original *Standards* was retained. The Committee believes that this revision is consistent with the guidance in the audit guide in all material respects. Significant changes and clarifications made within that framework follow:

General

1. *Voluntary health and welfare organizations* have been better defined.
2. Material in Chapter II of the previous edition, "Accounting Standards for Uniform Public Reporting," has been combined into other chapters where appropriate.
3. Outdated terminology related to United Ways and federated fund-raising organizations has been replaced.

Statement of Revenue, Expenses and Changes in Fund Balances

4. Examples and guidance on reporting *accounting changes* and *extraordinary items* in the financial statements have been added to the text. (p. 21–22)
5. The definitions of different types of transactions included in *Other Changes in Fund Balances* have been expanded. (pp. 21–22)
6. The primary-purpose rule for treatment of joint costs of informational materials and activities that include a fund-raising appeal is replaced with guidance on allocation of such costs as set forth in the AICPA Statement of Position 87-2. (pp. 54–57)
7. The word "support" is deleted from the title of the statement. (p. 16)

Balance Sheet

8. When appropriate, building campaign pledges are to be reported as deferred credits in the balance sheet until the date they are due. This is now consistent with practices previously followed for other types of pledges. (p. 26–27 and 74)
9. The circumstances under which *fund-raising expenses* may be deferred have been clarified. (p. 69 and 105–106)
10. The *columnar balance sheet* is presented as the primary format for the balance sheet. Other financial statements have been revised. (pp. 86–91)
11. The need for *capitalization of interest* in certain circumstances is recognized. (p. 72)

Other Changes

12. Appendix 6 on financial ratios has been added. (p. 121)
13. Guidance from SOP 78-10 on *combining of financial statements* of related organizations is included. (p. 79–83)
14. The Statement of Functional Expenses has been expanded to include Payments to the National Organization. (p. 91)
15. A brief note on Reporting of Service Efforts and Accomplishments has been added as Appendix 7. (p. 126)

CHAPTER II

RECOGNIZING "FUNDS" IN ACCOUNTING AND REPORTING

Much of the revenue received by voluntary agencies has no external restrictions on its use. These unrestricted funds can be used by the organization for any purposes designated by the governing board consistent with its charter and by-laws or mission. However, many such organizations also receive resources which are restricted for particular purposes or for use in locations specified by the donors. An agency may use a donor-restricted contribution only by complying with the terms of the donor's restriction. Only if the terms of an endowment instrument provide for eventual lifting of the restriction on the principal can the agency use the principal of the endowment gift for any other purpose, and then only after the removal of the restriction has occurred. Agency boards may also set aside, or designate, unrestricted funds for specified projects, as discussed below. However, since the board may change the designation, amounts designated by the board should not be included with donor-restricted, endowment, or land, building and equipment Funds, and the term "restricted" should not be used in connection with them.

As an agency receives increasing numbers of restricted gifts, these gifts may accumulate to the point of posing problems in maintaining a clear indication of the degree to which the donors' restrictions have been satisfied. One of the most important functions of a voluntary agency's public financial reporting is to show clearly that this is being accomplished.

THE NEED FOR THE "FUND" CONCEPT

The use of funds in accounting evolved from the need for orderly accounting and reporting on amounts restricted for different purposes. A Fund is a separate accounting entity with a self-balancing set of accounts for recording assets, liabilities, fund balance, and changes in fund balance. One of the distinctive characteristics of a Fund is that it is established to relate to the wishes and restrictions of the contributor.

Because of the restrictions associated with certain Funds, the financial statements should reflect unrestricted and restricted Funds separately. All unrestricted resources committed to or currently available for use in carrying out the organization's program and supporting services (except for unrestricted amounts invested in land, buildings and equipment, which may be accounted for in a separate Fund) should be segregated from those that are restricted as to use by the donor, by law or by other external authority.

The board may designate (such designations have at times been referred to as appropriations or allocations) portions of the Current Unrestricted Fund for various purposes as an aid in the planning of expenses and the conservation of assets. The organization may wish to maintain separate accounts for such designations within the Current Unrestricted Fund, and to segregate the designated and undesignated portions of the Fund on the balance sheet within the Fund balance section of the Current Unrestricted Fund.

Alternatively, when a columnar format is used to present the financial statements, the undesignated and board-designated portions of the Current Unrestricted Fund may be presented side by side provided a total Unrestricted Fund column is also presented. The three columns should be linked with an umbrella caption clearly disclosing that all the amounts presented are unrestricted.

Stewardship of Restricted Contributions

The agency that never receives gifts restricted to purposes and/or places specified by their donors escapes some real accounting problems. All contributions may be recorded in a single unrestricted Fund account. Any and all of the agency's bills may be met without considering restrictions by external authority.

Suppose, however, that an agency receives a contribution (Gift X) the donor wants used only for heart research. To assure that the money will not be considered unrestricted, a separate account is opened for the contribution in the general ledger. Then another contribution is received (Gift Y) "just for heart research." Does this require another new ledger account? No, the new gift may be recorded in the same account with the other.

Then, suppose the agency board decides to designate an amount for heart research from its unrestricted fund balance. The two Gifts, X and Y, are restricted by donors. They may therefore be combined in one ledger account, but only as restricted funds. The designated amount must be accounted for separately, since it represents board-designated unrestricted funds. The problem becomes even more difficult if yet another donor makes a contribution (Gift Z) for "only heart research" in a place. The gift has a double restriction (purpose and place) and it may be commingled with Gifts X and Y only if the place they will be used is the same as specified for Gift Z.

Reporting Restricted Contributions and Board-Designated Allocations

Gifts X, Y and Z are reported in the Current Restricted Fund column of Statement of Revenue and Expenses and Changes in Fund Balances—Exhibit B in the year of receipt. Expenses chargeable to the gifts are reported in the year they are incurred in the same column of Exhibit B. Any unexpended balance would be reflected in the Current Restricted Fund balance on the bottom line of Exhibit B and the Fund balance of Exhibit A. In the event Gift X or Y is only partly expended and, for some reason, the remaining funds are no longer required, it may be necessary, pursuant to the terms of the gift, to refund the unexpended balance to the donor. This refund (if made in a subsequent year) would be reported in Exhibit B in the Other Changes in Fund Balances section.

Board-designated funds are identified by segregating a part of the Current Unrestricted Fund balance on the Balance Sheet—Exhibit A. The board designations normally do not appear in Exhibit B, although there may be circumstances when this is desirable. However, expenses applicable to them will be included with other unrestricted Fund expenses in Exhibit B, in the Current Unrestricted Fund column. When these expenses are incurred, the amount of the board-designated funds in Exhibit A should be correspondingly reduced. If any remaining board-designated funds are no longer needed, as decided by the governing board, then the amount reflected in the designated Current Unrestricted Fund balance should be transferred to the undesignated, available for general activities classification of the Unrestricted Fund balance, or to some other designated unrestricted category as decided by the Board.

How far should an agency go in setting up separate accounts for restricted gifts, endowments, board designations or any other funds for which someone might be entitled to a detailed accounting? What rules should it follow in reporting transactions in separate Funds? The next discussion defines Funds for use by voluntary health and welfare organizations.

FUND ACCOUNTING IN REPORTS AND IN PRACTICE

Due to the various types of voluntary organizations and the variety of donor restrictions, the potential for creation of specific funds is almost unlimited.

To facilitate uniformity, the following Fund groups are recommended for standardized Fund reporting by voluntary health and welfare organizations:

Current Unrestricted Fund
Current Restricted Fund
Land, Building and Equipment Fund
Endowment Fund
Custodian and Other Funds

Current Unrestricted Fund

The Current Unrestricted Fund includes resources over which the governing board has discretionary control. It is used to account for resources which are available to carry out the purposes of the organization in accordance with the limitations of its charter and by-laws, except for unrestricted amounts invested in land, buildings and equipment accounted for in a separate Fund.

The principal sources of unrestricted funds are contributions, bequests, program service fees, dues, investment income, income from endowment funds, and sales of goods and services. Decreases in unrestricted funds generally result from expenses incurred for program services (including grants and allocations) and supporting services conducted by the organization. As discussed earlier, the board may designate portions of these resources for various purposes.

Current Restricted Fund

The Current Restricted Fund accounts for those resources currently available for use, but expendable only for operating purposes or in geographical locations specified by the donor or grantor. Such resources may originate from gifts, grants, income from endowment funds restricted for specific purposes, or other similar sources. Note that resources unrestricted as to purpose or place, but which are specified by the donor for use in a certain fiscal year, are reported in the current unrestricted fund. Accounting for such amounts is discussed on page 17–18 and 74.

"Specified by the donor or grantor" are the definition's key words. When contributors, rather than the governing board or the management of an agency, specify that their contributions are to be used only in a certain manner, the trust responsibility needs to be recognized by an agency in its accounts of the Current Restricted Fund for each distinct donor-specified purpose. Thus, this fund may include any number of donor-specified gifts, each of which must be controlled and accounted for in terms of amount received, expenses and Fund balances.

In contrast to the treatment accorded board designations, the Balance Sheet (Exhibit A) includes a separate, self-balancing section, in effect, a separate balance sheet for the assets, liabilities and Fund balances of the Current Restricted Fund. The segregation gives recognition to the fact that donor-restricted contributions must be used only for donor-specified purposes, and shows the assets available to fulfill commitments to the contributors.

Exhibit B, Statement of Revenue and Expenses and Changes in Fund Balances, makes this same distinction by showing current donor-restricted contributions, investment income, etc. in a separate restricted column.

The similarity of board designations and restricted gifts makes it advisable for agencies to minimize possibilities of confusion between the two by having the restrictions applying to significant restricted gifts stated in writing over the donor's signature. Word-of-mouth restrictions should be confirmed in writing. Amounts received from appeals for specific purpose(s) by solicitation letter, radio, television, newspaper, and so forth are generally deemed to be restricted according to the reason stated in the appeal.

Land, Building and Equipment Fund

The Land, Building and Equipment Fund (also referred to as the Plant Fund) is often used to accumulate the net investment in fixed assets and to account for the unexpended resources contributed specifically for the purpose of acquiring or replacing land, buildings or equipment for use in the operations of the organization. Mortgages or other liabilities relating to these assets are also included in this Fund.

The Fund balance of this Fund is divided into two categories in Exhibit A, expended and unexpended-restricted. The expended equity in fixed assets Fund balance reflects the net investment in fixed assets; unexpended-restricted reflects the balance of resources contributed but not yet expended. The portion of Current Unrestricted Funds designated by the governing board for the acquisition of fixed assets is not reported in the Land, Building and Equipment Fund, but is reported in the Current Unrestricted Fund balance of the Balance Sheet.

When new fixed assets, additions or replacements are acquired for agency use, regardless of the source of financing, these fixed assets, additions or replacements should be added to the Land, Building and Equipment Fund. Thus, in the case of fixed assets acquired with Unrestricted Fund resources, the amount expended should be reported as a transfer from the Current Unrestricted Fund to the Land, Building and Equipment Fund. On the other hand, proceeds from the sale of fixed assets formerly used in an agency's operations, and not legally required to be reinvested in fixed assets and with no restrictions on them should be transferred to the Current Unrestricted Fund. Such transfers should be reported in Exhibit B, Statement of Revenue and Expenses and Changes in Fund Balances, under Other Changes in Fund Balances. Gains or losses on the sale of fixed assets of the Land, Building and Equipment Fund should be reflected as part of other revenue in that Fund's column in Exhibit B. Chapters V and VI include an explanation of depreciation and its presentation in the operating statements and balance sheet.

Endowment Fund

The Endowment Fund accounts for the principal amount of gifts and bequests accepted with the donor stipulation that the principal be maintained intact in perpetuity, until the occurrence of a specified event or for a specified period, and that only the income from investment thereof be expended either for general purposes or for purposes specified by the donor.

If stipulated by the donor, investment income may accumulate in the Endowment Fund until the occurrence of a specified event, for a specified period, or until the balance reaches a specified level. Unless so stipulated, however, amounts are reported as income of the Current Unrestricted Fund or the Land, Building and Equipment Fund (see below). Net gains or losses from the sale of the investments or other property of this Fund should be accounted for in this Fund.

The principal of an endowment—the amount donated for investment—is to be reported, in the year of receipt, in the appropriate public support category of the Endowment Fund column of Exhibit B. The balance sheet includes a separate self-balancing section for the assets, liabilities and Fund balances of the Endowment Fund, thus recognizing the restrictions on them stipulated by the donors.

Therefore, it follows that income (as opposed to capital gains) earned on endowment investments may be either unrestricted, and therefore require no differentiation from other current investment income of an agency, or be donor-restricted, in which case the income is treated as restricted revenue. If endowment income is not donor-restricted, it should be credited, as earned, to investment income of the Current Unrestricted Fund. (Note that such income is *not* recorded first in the endowment fund and then transferred to the appropriate current fund.)

A voluntary agency that has endowment money invested in depreciable income- producing assets has a special depreciation problem. The necessity of preserving an endowment's principal intact (as is generally the case) requires that depreciation be charged as an expense against the related revenue; only the net income or loss after depreciation is available for distribution. In an agency's Exhibit B, the depreciation will be deducted from related rental income (and thus not affect the expenses section). In the balance sheet, accumulated depreciation should be treated the same way as it is for other depreciable assets, although the related assets in this case will be reported in the Endowment Fund.

Transfers from the Endowment Fund to other Funds are necessary in certain situations, e.g., lapsing of a term Endowment Fund restriction. In such a case, investment assets of the Endowment Fund are released. They should then be transferred and recorded by the recipient Fund at current market value. These transfers are reported under Other Changes in Fund Balances of Exhibit B. Any gain or loss (realized or unrealized) resulting from the adjustment in the current market value is recognized by the Fund making the transfer. [See Appendix 4. See also the discussion in Chapter IV of the transfer of a portion of gains on endowment investment.]

Custodian Fund and Other Funds

The Custodian Fund accounts for assets received by an organization to be held for, and disbursed only on instructions of, the person or organization from whom they were received.

Since custodian funds are not owned by the organization, the receipt of such funds or the income that might be generated from them should not be considered as a part of the organization's support or revenue. However, inclusion of the assets in the balance sheet requires that the assets be offset by a corresponding liability.

If other funds are significant, they should be accounted for separately. In many organizations the Annuity Fund is becoming more significant due to planned or deferred giving programs. Further, state laws may require the segregation of annuity funds from other funds.

Annuity and life income funds consist of funds acquired by an agency subject to agreements whereby assets are made available to the agency on the condition that the agency bind itself to pay the income earned thereon or other stipulated amounts periodically to designated individuals. Payments of such amounts terminate at a time specified in the agreements.

In many jurisdictions the "selling" or acceptance of annuities by a nonprofit organization is subject to the regulations of the appropriate governmental department or agency. Annuities can be issued only under regulations promulgated by the agency and, in some instances, investments of the annuity funds must be deposited or a security deposit made with the governmental jurisdiction. The supervising agency may also designate the types of investments which may be made with these funds.

Upon termination, the principal of these funds is transferred at current market value to the fund designated by the grantor or, in the absence of such a designation, to the Current Unrestricted Fund.

The actuarial method of recording annuity gifts requires the recording of the assets at cost or at fair market value at date of receipt. When a gift is received, the present value of the annuity payable, based upon acceptable life expectancy tables, is credited to a liability account and the remainder to revenue of the appropriate fund. Investment income and gains are credited, and annuity payments and investment losses are charged, to the liability account. Periodically, an adjustment is made to the liability to record the actuarial gain or loss due to recomputation of the liability based upon the revised life expectancy.

The statements of annuity funds are usually combined with those of life income funds, but each may be presented separately if significant. The sample financial statement in Exhibits A and B do not include such funds because for most agencies they are not significant.

CHAPTER III

THE OPERATING STATEMENTS

Contributors and others concerned with the financial needs and management of charitable organizations are interested primarily in the support an agency receives from different sources, and what it does with it—i.e., the expenses of operating the agency's service programs and other activities. The operating statement formats developed for uniform financial reporting by voluntary health and welfare organizations are presented in Chapter VIII: Exhibit B, Statement of Revenue and Expenses and Changes in Fund Balances* and Exhibit C, Statement of Functional Expenses. The statements are illustrative, as explained in that chapter, and it is not expected that all agencies will require the same number of classifications, since operations differ from agency to agency.

A brief review of these statements indicates that they differ from the formats of operating statements in general use by commercial organizations. This chapter will discuss the format of each of the exhibits and the reasons behind it.

Many organizations also prepare special reports for purposes other than public reporting. An example is the special project report which organizations submit to funding agencies (government agencies, foundations, etc.) to account for funds received for particular programs.

These reports vary considerably in format and content, depending on the funding agency's requirements, from a simple listing of support and/or revenue and expenses to detailed printed forms, such as those often specified by government agencies. In some instances, a funding agency may require an organization to prepare a special report pursuant to specified accounting procedures that may be at variance with generally accepted accounting principles. For example, a funding agency may require that the special report be prepared on a cash basis.

Due to the variety of special report formats that organizations may be required to comply with, this book will only address reporting in accordance with generally accepted accounting principles.

*In earlier editions of this book, this statement was called the "Statement of *Support*, Revenue, and . . ." The word "Support" has been dropped following the conclusion of the FASB in Statement of Financial Accounting Concepts (SFAC) 6 that support is part of revenue.

EXHIBIT B, STATEMENT OF REVENUE AND EXPENSES AND CHANGES IN FUND BALANCES

The first part of Exhibit B presents public support, revenue and grants from governmental agencies, other revenue, expenses and results of operations for each of the four primary Fund groups defined in Chapter II, the Current Unrestricted Fund; Current Restricted Fund; Land, Building and Equipment Fund; and Endowment Fund. The second part comprises Other Changes in Fund Balances for each of these Funds, i.e., interfund transfers and any other direct increases or decreases of the Fund balances during the year, the Fund balances at the beginning of the year, and the Fund balances at the end of the year. Agencies are required to report all their public support, revenue, expenses and other changes in Fund balances applicable to the year of the report in this statement. Generally, revenues are reported by source and expenses are reported by function. Each of the major sections of Exhibit B is discussed below.

Public Support Section

This section is divided into two parts: public support received directly and public support received indirectly. The term "public support"—comprising contributions of various kinds, special events, legacies and bequests, amounts received from federated and nonfederated fund-raising campaigns, etc.—represents charitable giving by the public in support of a voluntary agency. By contrast, the items grouped under other revenue comprise amounts earned by an agency through dues, fees, sales, investments and other income-producing activities. The revenue and grants from governmental agencies classification includes support and revenue from only one source: governmental agencies.

Donations from the public usually constitute the major source of public support for voluntary health and welfare organizations. Whether received directly as an unrestricted gift, a restricted gift for operating purposes, a restricted gift for the acquisition of fixed assets, an endowment (the income from which provides operating revenue), or indirectly received through an agency which provides fund-raising services for participating organizations, support is essential to the continuity of the organization.

While most support is in the form of cash, other means of making a contribution may be used. Thus, as further explained in Chapter IV, contributions may take the form of donated services, property, equipment and materials, which should be valued and included in support if certain criteria are met.

However, if donations (including pledges) received during the year are specified by the donor for use in future periods, these amounts should be initially recorded as deferred credits in the balance sheet of the appropriate Fund, and recorded as public support only in the year in which they may be used. In the absence of clear evidence as to a specified year or pledge payment schedule, donations and pledges should be recorded as public support in the year that notification of the pledge is received by the agency. Pledges with scheduled payments are often associated with a capital building campaign. Accordingly, these pledges should be assumed to be support in the periods of scheduled receipt, and should be initially accounted for as deferred credits on the balance sheet.

When recording pledges payable over more than one year, there might be a question regarding the propriety of recording the receivable at a discounted amount, reflecting assumed opportunity costs associated with the pledge collection period. The general practice in this situation is not to discount the pledge receivable, since receipt of a pledge is a nonreciprocal transaction, i.e., there has been no outlay of consideration by the beneficiary of the pledge, so there have been no opportunity costs incurred.

Public Support Received Directly

This subdivision of support received from the public is to be used to report all support received by an agency as a result of its own efforts—i.e., not through another organization. This would include grants and voluntary contributions received from individuals, corporations, and foundations.

Public Support Received Indirectly

Segregation of public support received indirectly, as shown in Exhibit B, results from the concern of many readers that they be able to relate fund-raising efforts to funds raised. Whenever possible, agencies should disclose parenthetically the fund-raising expenses incurred by the other organization associated with public support received indirectly. This requires that the other organization be contacted and that the necessary information be requested so that the reader may have a more complete understanding of the overall costs incurred in generating total public support. Segregation of indirect support as shown in Exhibit B accomplishes two objectives:

1. It points up separately the public support received directly by an agency through its own efforts or those under its direct supervision.
2. The reader is placed on notice by both the grouping and by the notes or parenthetic references to the associated fund-raising expenses, that fund-raising expenses incurred by the distributing organization and associated with indirect public support are netted against related support prior to distribution. Consequently, in Exhibit B, the fund-raising expenses shown

under supporting services represent primarily expenses incurred in obtaining public support received directly.

Revenue and Grants from Governmental Agencies

The number of Federal and other governmental agencies that grant funds to health and welfare organizations to carry out programs for which the agencies are responsible, or pay them fees for services rendered, makes it desirable to report this source of funding as a separate classification.

Other Revenue

Standardization of accounting and financial reporting by voluntary health and welfare agencies clearly requires that the concept of other revenue be applied with some precision. As mentioned previously, such revenue represents amounts earned and includes various types:

1. Gross revenue (without deduction of any costs or expenses) from program service activities—e.g., dues and fees for services and sales of program publications to the public. Related costs should be reported as program expenses.
2. Gross revenue from sales activities that are not a direct part of a major program but still relate to the organization's exempt purpose (not including direct personal services to individual patients and clients), or from sales of publications and materials to affiliated organizations and others. In some cases, it may be appropriate to report such revenues net of direct costs (such as printing and mailing costs for publications sold to affiliates), which should be disclosed parenthetically.
3. Investment income, gains and losses on investment transactions and other nonservice and nonsales related revenue. Note that some nonservice, nonsales types of revenues may be from profit generating activities unrelated to the exempt purpose of the organization. This "unrelated business income" is subject to taxation if the revenue-generating activities meet certain criteria established in the Internal Revenue Code, and generally should be reported net of related expenses.

Exhibit B reports revenue from program services as Other Revenue and costs of these services as program expenses.

Expense Section

The expense section includes all of an agency's expenses except certain direct costs of the types discussed above. First are the amounts spent by an agency in providing the services for which it has been organized and exists—i.e., the expenses of program services. The functional expense categories for program services will vary from one organization to another, depending upon the type of services rendered. For some organizations, a single program service category may be adequate to indicate the services provided. The second classification contains the expenses an agency incurs to provide the administrative and fund-raising services that support and make possible its program services—i.e., the expenses of its supporting services.

A third expense classification covers payments to affiliated organizations for unspecified purposes—e.g., those by local organizations to state/national affiliates. These payments will normally be used by the recipient affiliate for program services, management and general, and fund-raising expenses, but it is generally not proper for the paying affiliate to make an allocation of such payments to specific expense captions. (See the discussion in Chapter V.)

The format of the expense section of Exhibit B was developed to present expense information as simply and concisely as possible. Accordingly, it shows the total expenses of individual program and supporting service functions on a functional basis and by fund. Typically, most of the functional expenses represent costs financed by the Current Unrestricted Fund and are therefore reported in that Fund column. Expenses may also appear in the column for the Current Restricted Fund. Depreciation on fixed assets held for use must be reported entirely in the Land, Building and Equipment Fund, since it represents a cost applicable to the use of fixed assets. Interest expense incurred on debt recorded in the Land, Building and Equipment Fund (i.e., mortgages payable, equipment notes, capital lease obligations, etc.) should normally be reported in the Current Unrestricted Fund.

Exhibit B, Statement of Revenue and Expenses and Changes in Fund Balances, derives its functional expenses from Exhibit C, Statement of Functional Expenses. Total expenses of each function as shown on Exhibit C equal the corresponding expenses on Exhibit B.

Also, note that depreciation expense shown in Exhibit C is reflected entirely, as mentioned earlier, in the Land, Building and Equipment Fund on Exhibit B. The expense amounts in the Fund are comprised of depreciation, as shown in Exhibit C, and, if appropriate, an additional amount included in Supporting Services-Fund Raising which represents the costs of raising contributions for the building fund.

Many contributors are also interested in the objects of an agency's expenses—how much it spent for salaries, for rent, for staff travel, etc. In reporting to the public, voluntary agencies should therefore also provide a statement showing the composition of their functional expense totals according to the immediate objects of the expenses. Exhibit C, Statement of Functional Expenses, has been designed for this purpose and is discussed in the last part of this chapter.

Accounting Changes and Extraordinary Items

Since these types of transactions are rare for not-for-profit entities, current applicable professional literature does not provide specific examples of how to report the effects of accounting changes or extraordinary items in financial statements of voluntary health and welfare organizations.* The example following the Other Changes in Fund Balances section of this chapter shows the suggested treatment of an extraordinary item and the cumulative effect of an accounting change.

Other Changes in Fund Balances Section

This section provides for the reporting of changes affecting Fund Balances other than public support, revenue, and expenses. There are only a few types of transactions that can be properly reported here. These are discussed below:

Changes That Do Not Affect Total Fund Balances (Interfund Transfers)

1. Probably the most common change is the transfer from a Current Fund to the Land, Building and Equipment Fund of resources that have been used to purchase fixed assets for agency operations. This includes direct purchases of fixed assets as well as principal payments on mortgages payable, capital lease obligations [as defined in Statement of Financial Accounting Standards No. 13] and other property-related debt in the Land, Building and Equipment Fund. Because resources of a Fund other than the Land, Building and Equipment Fund were used, it is necessary to transfer an amount equal to these resources to the Land, Building and Equipment Fund from the Current Unrestricted and/or Current Restricted Funds.
2. Another type of transfer between the Current Unrestricted Fund and the Land, Building and Equipment Fund represents the transfer of proceeds from sales of fixed assets. The disposal of a fixed asset will normally result in the receipt of cash or establishment of a receivable. The proceeds (cash and/or receivable) should be reported as a transfer to the Current Unrestricted Fund.
3. Another type of transfer that would properly be shown in this section is the transfer to the Current Unrestricted Fund of part or all of the gains, as legally appropriate, on endowment funds. This is further discussed in Chapter IV.
4. A fourth type of transfer to be reported in Other Changes in Fund Balances is the transfer that needs to be made from the Endowment Fund to the appropriate Fund—e.g., Current Unrestricted Fund—when the restrictions

*Accounting Principles Board (APB) opinion No. 20 (reporting and accounting requirements for accounting changes), APB opinions No. 9 and No. 30 (extraordinary items), and SFAS No. 16 (prior period adjustments).

on a term endowment lapse and the related investment assets are released, as explained in Chapter IV and Appendix 4. Similar transfers would be made from annuity or life-income funds when the principal becomes legally available to the agency.

Changes That Do Affect Total Fund Balances

5. A fifth type of change in the Fund balance is the return to the donor of part or all of a restricted contribution. This occurs when a contribution is made, and either the donor requests a refund (an unlikely event), or an unexpended balance remains after all the conditions of the contribution are met and a refund is required. Note that any contribution refund made in the same accounting period in which the specific public support was recognized should be offset against public support. Only a refund of public support which had been recognized in a prior period should be reported as a change in Fund balance.

Example of Reporting Special Situations and Other Changes in Current Unrestricted Fund Balances

Excess of revenue over expenses before extraordinary items and cumulative effect of a change in an accounting principle	$XXX
Extraordinary items	XXX
Cumulative effect on prior years of a change in an accounting principle	XXX
Excess of revenue over expenses before other changes in Fund balances	XXX
Fund balances, beginning of year	XXX
Other Changes in Fund Balances:	
Property and equipment acquisitions from Unrestricted Fund	(XXX)
Transfer of proceeds from sales of fixed assets	XXX
Fund balances, end of year	$XXX

Due to the fact that accounting changes and extraordinary items occur infrequently in not-for-profit organizations, Exhibit B does not illustrate those special situations.

Fund Balances, Beginning of Year

Normally, these amounts will always agree with the ending fund balances of the prior period. Only in unusual circumstances would the beginning Fund balance amounts be restated. Restatement of the beginning Fund balance is required for a material prior-period adjustment which represents the correction of an error in prior years, and those few accounting principle changes which require restatement, typically resulting from issuance by FASB of pronouncements on matters not previously covered.

Fund Balances, End of Year

These are the final amounts shown on Exhibit B. They show the amounts at the end of the year in the four Fund balances and reflect the four respective Fund balances at the beginning of the year and all financial activity for the year. These amounts must, of course, agree with the corresponding amounts on Exhibit A—Balance Sheet.

Expanding the Detail of Exhibit B

For uniformity and comparability in financial reporting to the public by voluntary health and welfare agencies, it is recommended that their financial statements be uniform in format as well as content. To the extent applicable to a given agency, the report format and captions shown in Exhibit B and the order of presentation should be adhered to. Explanatory material provided in parenthetic notes in Exhibit B and in other financial statements, as well as in Notes to Financial Statements (Chapter VIII), must be adapted, of course, to the requirements of particular agencies. Some agencies may want to expand particular items of public support, other revenue, and expenses. For instance, revenue and grants from governmental agencies might be expanded as follows:

Revenue and grants from governmental agencies:	
Fees for services:	
City and county agencies	$XXX
State agencies	XXX
Total fees	XXX
Grant for child care cost study	XXX
Total revenue and grants from governmental agencies	$XXX

As long as the proper description and corresponding total of the expanded captions are shown, amplification of the exhibit is quite acceptable.

EXHIBIT C, STATEMENT OF FUNCTIONAL EXPENSES

Exhibit C has been designed to help those reading the financial statements of a voluntary agency to obtain a general understanding of the kinds of expenses included in each functional expense category shown in Exhibit B. Exhibit C reflects for each function the associated object expense categories—e.g., salaries, telephone, etc.

The number of object expense classifications has been purposely limited. Exhibit C is designed to present the major types of expenses included in each functional category, while avoiding burdensome detail. The detail shown in the statement will vary from one organization to another. The statement should, however, contain sufficient detail to enable the reader to gain a general understanding of the nature of the costs of carrying out the organization's activities. The level of detail shown in Exhibit C would generally provide this understanding.

Chapter V includes a section that describes the particular expenses included in each of the object expense categories illustrated in Exhibit C. Compilation of functional expense totals acceptable for reporting to the public requires that agencies apply rational methods of functional allocation to individual expenses, or types of expenses. (Appendix 1 is devoted to methods of allocation of expenses among functions.) Exhibit C requires that all costs related to building occupancy be included in occupancy, all costs related to travel in travel, etc. (See cost groupings in Chapter V.)

CHAPTER IV

THE CLASSIFICATION AND REPORTING OF PUBLIC SUPPORT AND OTHER REVENUE

This chapter deals in detail with the forms of public support and other revenue incorporated in Exhibit B. The arrangement of the classifications in Exhibit B is discussed in the preceding chapter. Public support and other revenue are to be reported in the financial statements in accordance with the appropriate classifications described below. This does not mean that agencies will require all the classifications and categories shown; rather, each agency should select from them those which adequately describe its support and other revenue.

Exhibit B, Statement of Revenue and Expenses and Changes in Fund Balances, provides for the reporting of support and other revenue in accordance with the stipulation of donors or other outside organizations, the reason stated in the fund-raising solicitation, or if no stipulations are expressed, as unrestricted. The format also provides for the reporting, by appropriate classifications, of total support received by the agency for all purposes.

PUBLIC SUPPORT RECEIVED DIRECTLY

Public support should be recorded in the accounts of the appropriate Fund—i.e., unrestricted support in the Current Unrestricted Fund; support restricted for specific operating purposes or places in the Current Restricted Fund; real estate, furnishings to be used by the organization, or funds contributed to acquire these or other fixed assets in the Land, Building and Equipment Fund; and support subject to restrictions of gift instruments, requiring that the principal be invested, in the Endowment Fund.

Public support received directly by an agency should be reported in its financial statements in accordance with the following classifications or subclassifications:

Contributions (subdivided by major source, if appropriate—i.e., individuals, corporations, foundations, etc.).
Special events.
Legacies and bequests.
Donated services, donated property, equipment and material.

Contributions

Contributions are to include only amounts received for which the donor derives no direct tangible benefits from the recipient agency. They are, therefore, to be distinguished from membership dues, program service fees, and special events, in which payments are made in return for tangible benefits.

All contributions received directly from individual donors and organizations, and not resulting from a federated fund-raising campaign, or the like, are to be included in this classification. Amounts paid ostensibly as memberships, but which are, in fact, contributions, and amounts paid in excess of the rate established as a regular membership, should be included here. (See the "membership dues—individuals" caption).

Illustrative of sources of support to be included in this category are the following:

Individuals.
Corporations and other businesses.
Foundations and trusts.
Contributors to door-to-door, mail and other solicitations conducted by an agency itself or by professional fund raisers or solicitors hired by the agency.
Fraternal, civic, social and other unrelated groups (direct contributions—excluding contributions raised through organized campaigns).
Also to be included in contributions are proceeds of special fund-raising activities other than "Special Events" which are discussed below.

As previously mentioned, the source of contributions—e.g., foundation grants—may be indicated in Exhibit B if desired. In those cases where amounts received from a specific source are significant in relation to the agency's total direct support, these amounts should be disclosed. Not to be included here, however, is support provided by governmental agencies or other support discussed in the following sections of this chapter.

Campaigns that voluntary agencies conduct to provide capital for major property additions—e.g., a building—require separate disclosure in Exhibit B. The reporting standards to be observed for uniform reporting to the public require that both the proceeds of these campaigns and the fund-raising expenses, provided the gifts to the capital campaign may be legally used to pay for fund raising, be reflected in Exhibit B in the Land, Building and Equipment Fund. The magnitude of these campaigns is likely to result in significant increases in both an agency's total contributions and total fund-raising expenses for a year in which a campaign was conducted. If not reported separately, this would preclude useful comparisons with results for other years or other agencies.

Contributions that are restricted for use in future accounting periods for the acquisition of land, buildings or equipment should be treated as deferred support in the Balance Sheet of the Land, Building and Equipment Fund. This is consistent with the treatment of other gifts restricted for use in future periods.

Special Events

The special events classification is provided to reflect support and incidental revenue—e.g., paid-for advertising in printed programs—derived from all of an agency's special fund-raising events during the period of the report. These are events in which something of tangible value is provided to donor participants or designees for a payment which includes a contribution adequate to yield revenue for the sponsoring agency over and above direct expenses. Support should also include the net proceeds received from raffled or auctioned items that have been donated or purchased. The value of items donated to an auction should not be included as a direct cost since the value received from the auction is really just a conversion of gifts in kind into cash. On the other hand, values of items donated to a raffle should be included as a direct benefit cost. Dinners, dances, bazaars, card parties, bingo, fashion shows, walk-a-thons, swim-a-thons, and cookie, candy and greeting card sales are examples of fund-raising activities which may qualify as special events. However, such activities may be included in the category only if the donors or designees receive a tangible benefit in return for payments. If no tangible benefit is received, the proceeds of the fund-raising activity should be included in the "contributions" category or shown in a separate caption.

The special event caption also discloses the cost of the direct benefits furnished to donor-participants or designees (see Exhibit B). The amount entered in the appropriate Fund column is to be the support remaining after deducting only the direct benefit costs. Direct benefit costs are defined as actual costs (not fair value to the recipient) to an agency of the dinner, ballroom, orchestra, decorations and refreshments in the case of a dance; of the price of admission to a theater party; of bazaar or circus prizes, etc.—i.e., the articles and services furnished as inducements directly to the participants.

All other direct and indirect expenses of promoting and conducting special events are to be reported directly as fund-raising expenses. Referred to here are such expenses as printing tickets and posters, mailings, fees and expenses of public relations and fund-raising consultants, other promotional activities, and the salaries and other expenses of the sponsoring agency itself that are reasonably allocable to the planning, promotion and conducting of special events.

To substantiate costs identified as direct benefits properly, an organization should maintain records for special events that show their gross proceeds separately from their direct costs.

The reporting described above applies only to special events sponsored by the reporting organization itself, or by an organization under its control. When a completely independent organization over which a voluntary agency has no control sponsors an event for the voluntary agency's benefit, the net proceeds received by the latter should be reported as contributions.

Special event support should be reported in the Fund which will benefit from the activity and which represents the purpose for which the special event was conducted (i.e., the Unrestricted Fund, unless the event was advertised as soliciting support for a particular purpose).

Telethons

Telethons and other forms of TV and radio entertainment are not usually considered special events for public reporting purposes. Contributions received in response to such appeals are normally to be reported as public support, and expenses attributable to the appeals as fund-raising expenses.

However, under certain conditions, a telethon or similar fund-raising event could have characteristics of a special event and thus warrant "special event treatment" in reporting on Exhibit B. To qualify as a special event, the above definition states that the fund-raising activity must demonstrate that "something of tangible value is offered directly to 'donor-participants' or designees for a payment and a contribution . . ." In a hypothetical situation, an agency could receive a payment for "something of tangible value" and a contribution from someone other than the participants (similar to the payment for advertising in a printed program). The fact that a payment would be made to cover all or part of the direct costs with benefit to the payor, in other words for "something of tangible value," will justify treating these costs, to the extent paid, as direct benefit expenses and permit their deduction from the gross received, with reporting of the net figure as explained later.

For example, an agency arranges to conduct a telethon. It commits itself for one and one-half hours of TV time at a cost of $75,000. A commercial company offers to sponsor one-half hour of the telethon by paying $25,000. The telethon raises $100,000 in contributions from TV viewers. The telethon in this situation warrants special event treatment on the Statement of Revenue and Expenses and Changes in Fund Balances. The gross amount received consists of $100,000 in contributions from TV viewers and $25,000 from the sponsor, or a total of $125,000. The direct benefit cost is the $25,000 paid by the sponsor for "something of tangible value" (for exposure gained by sponsoring one-half hour of TV time). This amount,

$25,000, is treated parenthetically on the Statement of Revenue and Expenses and Changes in Fund Balances as in the case of the usual form of special event. The net amount, $100,000, would appear on the telethon income line of the appropriate Fund column. The remaining $50,000 of the cost of the TV time, as well as all other fund-raising costs, would be included in expenses as part of the fund-raising function.

Whenever public support from telethons and similar fund-raising efforts is significant, it should be reported as a separate element of direct public support.

Legacies and Bequests

This category is to be used to report all legacies and bequests. A legacy or bequest is a gift made through a will or a living trust at the donor's death. Thus, gifts to be reported in this classification are those passing to the ownership of an agency by will or trust document after the death of the donor. The amount to be reported as legacy and bequest income should be net of legal and brokerage fees, taxes and other direct expenses incurred in clearing the agency's title to the gift or in converting the bequest to cash.

Legacies or bequests may be unrestricted or they may be restricted by the donor for specific purposes—i.e., fixed assets, geographic locations or for endowment. They should be reported in the Fund which is to be benefited. They should be reflected in the accounts of the agency only at the time that an unassailable right to the gift has been established by the probate court and the proceeds are measurable in amount.

Since legacies and bequests are received unpredictably, they generally cannot be related to the fund-raising efforts and expenses of an agency in any given year. Nevertheless, many organizations actively seek gifts through legacies and bequests, and some spend substantial sums in doing so. Further, these gifts are often substantial in size. Both their unpredictability and their potential size make it desirable that legacies and bequests be set forth separately by all agencies to facilitate evaluation of an agency's other contributions.

Many agencies receive income from trusts not under the control of the agency. A testamentary trust is a trust created by will; accordingly, the income from such a trust should be included with legacies and bequests. Income from other types of trusts should be included in contributions. If material, the income from trusts might be shown as a separate item in Exhibit B, and the existence, size and nature of the trust should be disclosed in the notes to the financial statements.

DONATED SERVICES, DONATED PROPERTY, EQUIPMENT AND MATERIALS

The services of unpaid volunteers and other noncash donations are resources sometimes more valuable to voluntary agencies than cash contributions. Free services of highly paid executives; contributions of material ranging from used typewriters to tracts of land; office space furnished rent-free; publicity donated by television, radio and other media—all raise the question: should they be valued and reported in an agency's financial statements? Uniform accounting and reporting of donated materials and services is further complicated by the diverse sources of this support. While it is usually possible for a local voluntary agency to request and receive from a national organization with which it is affiliated, realistic values for services and materials furnished free of charge by the national to the local, voluntary agencies may well encounter very real problems in attempting to evaluate noncash donations from individuals and organizations from whom they have no right to demand any kind of accounting. This part of the chapter will consider standards of accounting and reporting for donations from organizations and individuals over whom the recipient agency has no real supervision or control, as well as those situations where the agency does have supervision and control.

Donated Personal Services

Voluntary agencies may benefit from independently donated services of many kinds, from fund raising by volunteers in neighborhood solicitations to the services of business executives. There are three accounting issues associated with donations of services by individuals or organizations. Would the services performed normally be purchased by an agency if volunteers were not available? What is a clearly measurable basis for assigning values to these services? How does the agency exercise control over the services offered—over the "who," "what," "when," and "how" of services—that determine their real value to an agency? Thus, in the case of the volunteers soliciting funds, an agency will rarely have any measurable basis for valuing the time spent. The same question arises in the case of the business executive who assumes a position of responsibility in the annual campaign of a United Way: a person's business earnings cannot necessarily be assumed to be a measure of value to a United Way campaign. Nor can it be supposed, in either case, that the benefited organization has sufficient control over all major elements of the services offered, nor that the services performed would otherwise be carried on by salaried personnel.

The difficulties just cited may explain the frequent omission from voluntary agencies' financial statements of any financial values for independently donated services. Nevertheless, in the interest of adequate disclosure to the public, it is considered necessary to adopt the rule that, where significant, donated services will be included in an agency's Statement of Revenue and Expenses and Changes in Fund Balances (Exhibit B) in the following circumstances:

1. The services performed are a normal part of the program or supporting services and would otherwise be performed by salaried personnel;
2. The organization exercises control over the employment and duties of the donors of the services; and
3. The organization has a clearly measurable basis for the dollar amount to be recorded.

Services which generally are not recorded as contributions, even though these services might constitute a significant factor in the operation of the organization, include:

1. Supplementary efforts of volunteer workers provided directly to beneficiaries of the organization. Such activities may comprise auxiliary activities or other specific services that would not otherwise be provided by the organization as a part of its operating program.
2. Periodic services of volunteers needed for concentrated fund-raising drives. The activities of volunteer solicitors are not usually subject to a sufficient degree of operating supervision and control by the organization to enable it to have a proper basis for measuring and recording the value of the time spent.
3. Professional personnel engaged by another organization in research and training activities with or without pay. This type of work, usually performed in connection with grants made by the organization to other agencies, universities or institutions for specific research projects, is not under the direct supervision and control of the granting organization, and normally the work is being done as part of the activities of the recipient institution rather than the granting agency. Accordingly, it is ordinarily considered not practicable to compute a value for these services.

The financial statements should disclose the amount of donated services and the methods followed by the organization in evaluating, recording and reporting donated services.

Donated Land, Buildings, Property, Equipment and Materials

Generally, donations of land, buildings and equipment should be recorded at their fair value at date of gift. Agencies that receive the use of a building partially or completely rent-free should report, as a contribution, the difference between the rent paid and the fair rental value of the space occupied to the extent objectively determinable. Objective fair rental values may be available, for instance, in the amount charged to the previous tenant in a building or office, or in going rental values for comparable space in the same area.

Donated Materials

Important differences exist among voluntary health and welfare organizations in the types of material donations that they solicit and accept, in the processing to which donated materials are subjected and in the ultimate uses of these materials. Sheltered workshops for training or employment of handicapped persons depend upon continuous solicitation and collection of discarded clothing, furniture and other household articles. Some health agencies receive costly drugs donated by pharmaceutical houses for use in their therapeutic programs. Agencies engaged in relief activities in developing countries or in disaster areas often solicit contributions of new, as well as used, equipment of various kinds. Agencies also receive gifts of items for their own use such as office equipment, vehicles, etc. Standardization of accounting is necessary not only for valuing materials received as contributions, but also for the costs of soliciting and collecting the materials and for their use, including processing and disposal costs, in an agency's activities.

Donated materials of significance should be recorded at their fair market value when received, if their omission would cause the Statement of Revenue and Expenses and Changes in Fund Balances to be misleading and if the organization has an objective, clearly measurable basis for the value, such as net proceeds from resale by the organization, price lists or market quotations (adjusted for deterioration and obsolescence) or appraisals. This recording is necessary not only to account properly for all transactions of the organization, but also to enhance stewardship control over all materials received.

If the nature of the materials is such that valuations cannot readily be substantiated, they should not be recorded as contributions; used clothing received as contributions and subsequently given away might, for example, fall into this category. There is, of course, no valuation problem where donated materials are converted into cash soon after receipt, since the net cash received is an acceptable gauge of the value of the contribution.

When donated materials are used in rendering the service provided by the organization, the cost of these materials included in the service is based on the value previously recorded for the contribution. If donated materials pass directly through the organization to its charitable beneficiaries with the organization merely serving as an agent for the donors, the donation would not normally be recorded as a contribution nor the distribution of the materials as an expense.

If significant amounts are involved, the value of the materials recorded as contributions and as expenses (or assets, if appropriate) should be clearly disclosed in the financial statements.

PUBLIC SUPPORT RECEIVED INDIRECTLY

This section discusses the following categories of Exhibit B under public support received indirectly:

Collected through local member units.
Contributed by associated organizations.
Allocated by federated fund-raising organizations.
Allocated by unassociated and nonfederated fund-raising organizations.

Collected Through Local Member Units

Some national health and welfare organizations derive major financial support from fund-raising campaigns conducted by their local affiliates for support of the national, as well as of the local organization. The proceeds of such a combined national-local fund-raising campaign are commonly allocated between the local agency and its national affiliate on the basis of a predetermined ratio. In these conditions, the national organization should report its share—in effect, public support derived through efforts of the local agency expressly on its behalf—in this classification and also, parenthetically, the fund-raising costs relative to its share, in the financial statements or notes.

Contributed by Associated Organizations

This classification is to be used to report contributions from auxiliaries, circles, guilds and other organizations closely associated with the reporting organization, but not for membership payments in the form of dues or assessments. Further, only contributions from organizations directly related to the recipient by identity of purpose, programs or clientele should be reported here. Contributions from a sponsoring "parent" agency or from sponsoring religious bodies would also be reported here, but not contributions from foundations, a local civic organization or other unrelated group. The estimated fund-raising costs in raising the contributions should be disclosed parenthetically.

Excluded from this classification, in addition, are contributions or allocations received from federated and other fund-raising organizations, including United Ways, and such sectarian organizations as the various Catholic Charities and Jewish Federations. Contributions received by an agency from these types of fund-raising organizations belong in one of the two categories described below.

Allocated by Federated Fund-Raising Organizations

All allocations, appropriations and other forms of financial support received or receivable from federated fund-raising organizations, as defined in Appendix 2, are to be reported in this classification. The name (or names) or type of the particular organization from which the support was received may be used in place of the term "federated fund-raising organization." In addition, the estimated fund-raising costs incurred by the other organization in raising the contributions should be disclosed parenthetically. The timing of recording of receivables and revenue should be the same as for public support received directly.

Allocated by Unassociated and Nonfederated Fund-Raising Organizations

This category is provided for reporting support derived from fund-raising campaigns received from specialized fund-raising organizations that are not associated with a reporting agency as previously described (in "Contributed by Associated Organizations" and "Allocated by Federated Fund-Raising Organizations"). This category is to be used to report allocations to an agency that result from independent nonfederated campaigns for multiple-agency support organizations. Here again, it is recommended that the specific sources be identified and shown in an agency's report.

REVENUE AND GRANTS FROM GOVERNMENTAL AGENCIES

All support and other revenue that an agency receives from governmental sources is to be reported in this classification. For some agencies, this may require the combining of purchase-of-services fees and contract payments from local, state and Federal organizations with research and other grants from these units. The importance to private agencies of government payments of all types and the frequent difficulty in classifying many types of payments unambiguously as either support or other revenue make it desirable to report the total of this support and revenue in a single figure in Exhibit B, rather than to classify the payments in support or other revenue, as the case may be. Agencies may differentiate among sources and kinds of governmental support in a separate schedule keyed to this classification in Exhibit B, Statement of Revenue and Expenses and Changes in Fund Balances, or sub-classifications may be used in the exhibit itself. (Many governmental grants are restricted to specific programs; such amounts would usually be reported in the Current Restricted Fund along with their related expenses.)

OTHER REVENUE

The other revenue section of Exhibit B comprises:

Membership dues—individuals.
Assessments and dues—local member units.
Program service fees and net incidental revenue.
Sales of materials and services to member units (Net of direct expenses).
Sales to the public.
Investment income.
Gains (or losses) on investment transactions, or sales of other assets.
Miscellaneous revenue.

Membership Dues—Individuals

As already noted, the Membership dues—individuals caption is reserved for amounts received by an agency for personal memberships that procure directly for the member tangible benefits commensurate in value with the amount of the dues. Substantial direct, private benefits may include: the use of agency recreational, consulting and other facilities and services; the right to participate in educational programs; the right to receive directly useful publications; or the enjoyment of a professional standing or other honor.

Voting rights alone are not sufficient to qualify a payment as a membership payment. Newsletters must, in many instances, also be rejected as an insufficient benefit to qualify a payment as a membership. If a newsletter-type publication has no other function than to keep a member informed of general activities of an organization, it would not normally be considered of sufficient direct tangible benefit to classify payments received from "members" in this category.

"Contributing," "sustaining" and similar memberships implicitly require scrutiny for proper reporting. Their distinguishing titles imply there is an alternative, "regular" membership with a difference in rates charged. If the regular membership, in fact, qualifies as a "time" membership, as just defined, and if the benefits offered for a "contributing" or "sustaining" membership are not in fact greater, corresponding to the difference in charge, then the difference between the charge collected and the rate for a regular membership properly is reported in contributions.

Revenue derived from membership dues should be recognized by the organization over the period to which the dues relate. Non-refundable initiation and life-membership fees should be recognized as revenue in the period the fees are receivable, if future dues or fees can reasonably be expected to cover the cost of future services; otherwise, the fees should be amortized to future periods based on average membership duration, life expectancy, or other appropriate methods. However, if items such as dues assessments and non-refundable initiation fees are, in substance, contributions—and services are not to be provided to the member—they should be recognized as contributions in the periods in which the organization is entitled to them.

Assessments and Dues—Member Units

Amounts received by an organization from its member agencies (at the local, state and regional levels, etc.) for general membership benefits are to be reported here. Use of the classification should be restricted to revenues from dues, fair share quotas and similar assessments against member agencies to cover regular services, publications, materials and other membership benefits furnished to all member agencies of the same class. As previously discussed, amounts received from fund-raising campaigns that solicit support for both the sponsoring agency and its national affiliate—the proceeds of which are divided between the two according to a predetermined formula—do not belong in this caption. Amounts received as fees for special consulting services to particular member agencies and revenue from sales of materials ordered by and billed separately to individual agencies should not be reported here, but should be shown under sales of materials and services to local member units.

Program Service Fees and Net Incidental Revenue

This classification includes two distinct types of revenue received from participants in an agency's programs. The first type are fees received for the agency's program services and other revenues from program-related activities. The second consists of the excess of revenues over expenses of service-related activities that are only incidental to the service. (Amounts received from governmental agencies and member agency payments for services to the agencies themselves are not to be reported here.) Either of the two types of revenue may appear alone in Exhibit B in the absence of revenue of the other type. Each will be considered separately.

Program Service Fees

This classification provides for fee payments, received either from the recipient or non-governmental third parties, for health and welfare services furnished by an agency. Whether an agency uses schedules of fees for different services or merely requests clients to pay what they feel they can afford, as in the case of many church-related agencies, any type of payments in return for an agency's professional services belong in this classification. Some agencies account for fees by recording them at established standard rates for services rendered, then apply "allowances" to reduce the standard to the amount actually charged in each case. Such agencies should report as program service fees only the net actually charged.

Whether a particular payment should be treated as program service fees or as a contribution may raise questions for some agencies. The individual asked to "contribute" whatever he thinks he can afford, in (partial) payment for an agency's services, may feel justified in reporting the payment on his income tax return as a contribution. This personal decision need neither affect nor depend upon the agency's public reporting of the payment.

Program Net Incidental Revenue

The second type of revenue to be included in program service fees is revenue from activities that, although administered by it, a voluntary agency regards as incidental to its primary services. Examples are: the excess of fees collected from participants in a "pay-your-own-way outing" over bus charter and other group expenses, some agency-sponsored student conferences, provision of display space to exhibitors at conventions, and neighborhood self-improvement projects sponsored by an agency but on the periphery of its primary social service programs.

Agencies generally attempt to make these activities self-supporting by charging registration fees, rentals and other service charges at rates intended to cover their direct expenses and, in some instances, properly allocable administration and other indirect expenses. Accordingly, the revenues and expenses of such activities are generally netted and the net revenues or expenses are included in the appropriate revenue or expense caption in Exhibit B.

Some of the program activities of sheltered workshops and other agencies that generate revenue will require careful review for correct classification. The expenses of revenue-producing activities that are conducted primarily as therapeutic training or for other program purposes should be grouped with an agency's program services in the expense section of Exhibit B. In the latter section, an excess of expenses over incidental revenue (sales activites related incidentally to therapeutic training) should appear as program-service expenses supported by general revenue. In the event that revenue from such activities exceeds expenses, the net revenue should be reported in the revenue section. In both cases, the amount deducted should be disclosed. (See also the discussion of reporting program-related income above.)

An exception to this last rule exists, however, with respect to fund-raising work performed by client-workers of a sheltered workshop. By definition, this work may not be regarded as a primary program service of an agency. Wages paid to client-workers for fund-raising work should be included with other fund-raising expenses of the sheltered workshop. Contributions resulting from their efforts are to be reported in full, on the other hand, under contributions.

Sales of Materials and Services to Member Units

This classification is provided for the revenue obtained by health and welfare organizations from sales to their member agencies of publications and materials, consultation and other services. In general, it should be used by a voluntary organization to report sales and special-service fees billed to an associated health or welfare agency. Royalties and other sales-based payments to national organizations by manufacturers, related to sales of insignia and other agency-identified materials directly to local agencies for resale to bona fide individual members, are also to be reported in this classification. The directly related expenses, shown in Exhibit B as deducted in arriving at the amount entered in the column, should be all direct costs of the materials and services reasonably allocable to them.

Sales to the Public

Sales of program-related publications and materials to the general public are to be segregated from sales to member agencies and reported gross. Related costs and expenses—e.g., printing and mailing—should be reported in the appropriate program expense category. However, sales of nonprogram-related items to the general public should be segregated from sales to member agencies and reported net of related expenses.

Investment Income

A voluntary health or welfare agency may earn income from a variety of investments, from securities held for long-term or short-term investment to real estate and patents acquired through gifts or bequests and retained by the agency. In form, investment income may include interest, dividends, rent, royalties and even net earnings from activities—e.g., operation of an office building acquired through an endowment conducted solely for the production of income. All investment income of whatever type or origin (other than capital gains, as discussed in the next section) is to be summarized and reported as investment income in Exhibit B.

Income on investments of unrestricted funds should be reported in investment income of the Current Unrestricted Fund. Income on investments of restricted funds, other than endowment funds, should also be included in investment income of the Current Unrestricted Fund, unless it is specifically restricted by the donor or legally required to be used for restricted purposes.

Investment income of an Endowment Fund, unless restricted to a specific purpose by terms of the gift instrument, is available for unrestricted purposes and should be included in investment income of the Current Unrestricted Fund. Where the donor has restricted the use of the income from the investment of the endowment gift, such income should be included in investment income of the Current Restricted Fund or other appropriate Fund. In both cases, the investment income should be reported directly in the appropriate fund and *not* in the Endowment Fund.

Gains (or Losses) on Investment Transactions and Sales of Other Assets

The net amount of gains or losses should be reported in gains (or losses) on investment transactions of Exhibit B, even if the net figure is a loss. If gains (losses) on sales of assets other than investments are significant, the amount should be separately disclosed. Gains or losses that derive from investments of unrestricted funds should be reported in the column for the Current Unrestricted Fund on Exhibit B.

Gains or losses on investments of restricted funds, other than endowment funds, should be included in gains (or losses) on investment transactions in the Current Unrestricted Fund, unless not legally available for unrestricted purposes, in which case they should be included in the same category of the Current Restricted Fund, or Land, Building and Equipment Fund, as appropriate.

A special procedure can apply to gains and losses on investment transactions of endowment funds. Prior to the 1970s, realized gains and losses on investments of endowment funds generally were considered as principal transactions, and all restrictions which pertained to the original corpus of the funds had been deemed to apply to the net realized gains—i.e., they were added to principal. Only when the endowment instrument specifically stated that such gains and losses were not so restricted, had these amounts been considered as income and available for operating purposes.

The statutes of several states now provide that certain nonprofit organizations subject to their jurisdictions may, in certain circumstances, consider net realized (and in some cases, unrealized) gains on investments of endowment funds as available for unrestricted use. The law of one state, for example, provides that the amount of such funds to be made available for unrestricted use may include so much of the realized appreciation of principal as the governing board may deem prudent, provided the amount of fair value of the remaining principal shall not be less than the fair value of the original assets at the time received. Under this approach, gains and losses are initially recorded in the Endowment Fund, as usual, then a portion of the realized (and in some cases, unrealized) capital appreciation in the Endowment Fund is made available for operating purposes, and assets equal to this amount are transferred to the Current Unrestricted Fund. The designated amount of appreciation to be transferred to the Current Unrestricted Fund should be reflected as a transfer in the other changes in Fund balances section of Exhibit B. Amounts of investment gains included in the Endowment Fund available for transfer to the Current Unrestricted Fund at the discretion of the governing board should be disclosed in the notes to the financial statements; the authority on which such funds may be transferred should also be disclosed.

Investment Pools—Allocation of Investment Income, Capital Gains and Losses

To obtain investment flexibility, voluntary health and welfare organizations frequently pool investments of various funds in a single investment program—e.g., a single portfolio of securities. The term "Funds" as used here refers to Fund entities in a broad sense. It includes not only any of the organization's structural Funds that can combine investments—the Current Unrestricted Fund; the Current Restricted Fund; the Land, Building and Equipment Fund—but also such other Funds as may have been established either by terms of a gift or legacy—e.g., William Johnson Memorial Fund—or by board action.

Because the realized and unrealized gains (losses) and income are not identified directly with the specific Funds participating in the pool, it is of paramount importance that realized and unrealized gains (losses) and income be allocated equitably. To accomplish an equitable allocation, investment pools should be operated on the market-value method. Under this method, each Fund is assigned a number of units based on the relationship of market value of all Funds at the time the investments are pooled. Periodically, the pooled assets are valued and new unit values assigned. The new unit value is used to determine the number of units to be allocated to new Funds entered in the pool or to calculate the equity of Funds withdrawn from the pool. Investment pool income should be allocated to participating Funds based on the number of units held by each Fund. In cases where the income of one or more of the participating Funds has been restricted by the donor for specified purposes, it may be necessary to account for gains and losses, due to market price changes, separately from other investment pool income—i.e., interest and dividends—since gains and losses may revert to the corpus of the restricted Fund.

An illustration of the operation of an investment pool can be found in Appendix 3.

Miscellaneous Revenue

This classification needs no explanation, but a word of caution may be appropriate. If the revenue of an agency has been properly classified, very little should usually remain to be shown as miscellaneous. Transactions that may be run through a suspense account can generally be designated, as they occur, for specific revenue and expense accounts. Many are recognizable as involving funds belonging to someone other than the agency and thus are custodian funds and in no sense revenue to the agency. They should not appear in Exhibit B at all. Others represent expense reimbursements that can be credited at once to specific expense accounts. The more frequently "suspense," "revolving," and similar catch-all accounts are used, and the longer they are left unattended, the more difficult it becomes to avoid accumulating unidentifiable entries and an undesirable large total of miscellaneous.

If significant, income from ongoing business activities unrelated to the agency's exempt purpose should be shown separately—net of related expenses.

Public Support and/or Revenue Allocable to National Programs (Deduction)

See payments to affiliated organizations in Chapter V (see p. 50–51).

CHAPTER V

THE CLASSIFICATION AND REPORTING OF EXPENSES

The operating statements described in Chapter III have been designed to satisfy three common concerns of contributors with respect to the expenses of a voluntary agency:

1. To see all of an agency's expenses reported with its support and revenue in a single statement (Exhibit B).
2. To see how much it spent on each of its program functions and supporting services (Exhibit B).
3. To see the distribution of object expenses—e.g., salaries, travel, printing—among its program functions and supporting services (Exhibit C).

Contributors, contributor information and budget review groups, regulatory bodies, and trustees and officials of voluntary agencies are most interested in the cost of the various services and other activities provided by health and welfare agencies. They want to know the cost to an agency of each of its program functions and the costs of fund-raising and management and general services. To satisfy these interests, Exhibit B, the operating statement designed for public reporting by voluntary health and welfare organizations, provides for functional reporting of expenses.

The first part of this chapter describes the two major functional classifications incorporated in Exhibit B, program services and supporting services. Supporting services are further subdivided into management and general and fund-raising. It also discusses the expense classification, "payments to affiliated organizations." Succeeding parts of the chapter examine the problems of classifying public education, public information and fund-raising information expenses, problems of calculating and comparing fund-raising ratios, and standardization of reporting of awards and grants made by an agency. The object expense groupings of Exhibit C are discussed in the chapter's last section.

Functional reporting of expenses according to the format of Exhibit B requires that agencies combine the expenses of particular activities according to their essential purposes—i.e., program, management and general, and fund raising. For example, an agency that recognizes operation of a summer camp as one of its distinct program functions should include in its reported camp program expenses the costs of infirmary, trading post and other auxiliary activities that are integral parts of the camping program. In some instances, it will be necessary to break down the salary of an individual among two or more program functions that the person serves—e.g., the salary of a staff physician between a camping program and the program services participated in during non-summer months. Other expenses, such as rent, materials and travel, will frequently need to be divided among the several functional purposes served. Methods of making such divisions, or allocations, are discussed in Appendix 1.

PROGRAM SERVICES

This first major expense designation in Exhibit B is a caption, or heading, under which an agency is to list its major health or welfare program service categories, the total expenses for each during the reporting period and the total of all program services.

Uniform, comparable expense reporting by voluntary agencies would be greatly advanced if it were possible to devise a satisfactory set of universal program service categories. These would have to be sufficiently definitive (as well as broad), however, to permit any agency, without distorting their significance, to fit all its program service expenses into one standard category or another.

Uniform Program Service Categories for Health Agencies

One group of voluntary agencies, the national voluntary health organizations that are members of the National Health Council, has used standard program classifications for almost thirty years. The program service classifications defined by the National Health Council for its voluntary member agencies comprise five functional expense categories:

Research
Public health education
Professional health education and training
Patient services
Community health services

These expenses are defined as follows:

> The research category represents awards or grants-in-aid to support scientific studies or investigations, plus all other costs or expenses incurred while conducting a program in which new knowledge is being sought to find causes, cures and prevention for specific diseases or health problems.
>
> The public health education category represents programs conducted for the purpose of informing the general public how to promptly recognize

the symptoms of ill health, disease and/or physical disorders. Also included is the dissemination of facts and information designed to encourage periodic physical examinations, reduce indifference toward health problems and eliminate unwarranted fears or misconceptions. All other costs or expenses directly related to the performance of "health" educational work also fall under this category.

The professional health education and training category represents activities or programs designed to improve the knowledge, skills and critical judgment of physicians, dentists, nurses and others engaged (directly or indirectly) in health work by keeping them abreast of new medical advancements, diagnostic techniques, etc. Also part of this category is the provision of educational opportunities for those who have displayed the interest, aptitude and intelligence to enter the medical field or undertake scientific investigations, as well as expansion or improvement of health educational courses in universities or the like and stimulation of health and/or scientific careers. In addition, all other costs or expenses incurred while endeavoring to enlarge the number and quality of medical personnel, and professional health workers, in general, would be included.

The patient services category represents activities performed or programs conducted for the purpose of providing physical, emotional and other assistance to individuals afflicted with a disease or health impairment, or to their families. The category further includes the furnishing of medical care, hospitalization, equipment, drugs and other tangible items to those in need, plus all other costs or expenses incurred as a result of assisting individuals while bedridden or physically incapacitated.

The community services category represents activities such as the detection of disease or health problems, planning and improving community health practices, supporting clinics or other public health facilities, conducting rehabilitative and similar programs. Also represented are all other costs or expenses incurred in performing functions, which, directly or indirectly, accrue to the community's benefit.

Status of Program Service Classifications Among Other Voluntary Agencies

It is highly desirable that a single set of program service categories be used by all the highly diverse health and welfare organizations in the United States. A significant aid in achieving this objective is the United Way of America Services Identification System, Second Edition [UWASIS II], A Taxonomy of Social Goals and Human Service Programs, published in 1976.

UWASIS II is a compendium of definitions of government and voluntary human service programs in the United States. UWASIS II outlines the basic social goals, the services systems which promote such goals, the specific services in such systems, the programs which perform such services, some elements of such programs, and suggested program products—in terms of types of persons served and efforts expended on their behalf. The system provides a conceptual framework for identifying, classifying, and defining most current human endeavors for dealing with human problems and aspirations. The areas of concern encompassed by UWASIS II range from employment, income maintenance, health, housing, education, and transportation to environmental protection, consumer protection, social development, and equal opportunity.

The broad social goals articulated in UWASIS II are:

I. OPTIMAL INCOME SECURITY AND ECONOMIC OPPORTUNITY
II. OPTIMAL HEALTH
III. OPTIMAL PROVISION OF BASIC MATERIAL NEEDS
IV. OPTIMAL OPPORTUNITY FOR THE ACQUISITION OF KNOWLEDGE AND SKILLS
V. OPTIMAL ENVIRONMENTAL QUALITY
VI. OPTIMAL INDIVIDUAL AND COLLECTIVE SAFETY
VII. OPTIMAL SOCIAL FUNCTIONING
VIII. OPTIMAL ASSURANCE OF THE SUPPORT AND EFFECTIVENESS OF SERVICES, THROUGH ORGANIZED ACTION

Thirty-three services systems, 231 services and 587 programs are identified, defined, and classified within the above 8 goals—a total of 859 titles, including most programs listed in the *Catalogue of Federal Domestic Assistance*, published by the U.S. Government.

Illustrative Program Service Definitions and Classifications

As previously indicated, functional expense reporting is a technique of accounting for expenses of activities that constitute a single service program. The usefulness of such accounting depends very much on the care with which an agency defines and relates its activities to functions. To furnish a practical basis for expense accounting, definitions of individual program services should include identification of expenses of particular activities exclusively with one program or another, to the greatest extent possible.

In defining its own service programs for uniform reporting to the public, as discussed previously in "Status of Program Service Classifications Among Other Voluntary Agencies," an agency should attempt to confine its program service classifications to the major functional purposes it serves and to those that exhibit practically distinguishable direct costs.

The following page is an illustration of how human service programs are organized under UWASIS II schema.

7.0.00.00

GOAL VII: OPTIMAL SOCIAL FUNCTIONING

7.1.00.00 INDIVIDUAL AND FAMILY LIFE SERVICES SYSTEM

7.1.01.00 **Family Preservation and Strengthening Service**

Programs

7.1.01.01 Counseling
7.1.01.02 Interventive Assistance to Mobile Families and Individuals
7.1.01.03 Comprehensive Family Life Education
7.1.01.04 Single-Parent Family Development
7.1.01.05 to 7.1.01.99 AIN—Family Preservation and Strengthening Service

7.1.02.00 **Family Substitute/Foster Care Service**

Programs

7.1.02.01 Adoption
7.1.02.02 Foster Family Care—Children
7.1.02.03 Foster Family Care—Adults
7.1.02.04 Group Home—Children
7.1.02.05 Group Home—Adults
7.1.02.06 Emergency Shelter Care—Children
7.1.02.07 Emergency Shelter Care for the Homeless and Transients
7.1.02.08 Institutional Care—Children
7.1.02.09 Institutional Care—Adults
7.1.02.10 Domiciliary Care for Veterans
7.1.02.11 Residential Care for Runaways
7.1.02.12 Residential Care and Supportive Assistance to Unwed Pregnant Females
7.1.02.13 to 7.1.02.99 AIN—Family Substitute/Foster Care Service

7.1.03.00 **Family Supplementing Service**

Programs

7.1.03.01 Day Care—Children
7.1.03.02 Day Care—Adults
7.1.03.03 Respite Care
7.1.03.04 Homemaker Assistance

Each individually identified program is defined in terms of various elements.

Reporting Income Related to Program Services

A logical sequel to accounting for expenses primarily by program services is to account for fees and other program-related income the same way—in order to determine the net cost of each of an agency's services. Invaluable as is such program-by-program matching of revenues and expenses for financial management of agencies, it is not necessarily appropriate for reporting to the public at large. For uniform financial reporting, voluntary agencies should normally report program service fees and related revenue as "program service fees and net incidental revenue," and program service expenses in an appropriate program service expense category.

SUPPORTING SERVICES

If diversity characterizes the program services reported by different types of voluntary agencies, all agencies can recognize certain uniform characteristics in the services that support their program services. These supporting services may be distinguished as being either management and general or fund raising in character.

Management and General

All organizations, whether business concerns, governmental bureaus or charitable organizations, carry on a variety of essential activities identifiable with no one of their primary functions but indispensable to the conduct of all of them and to an organization's corporate existence. It is an agency's expenses for these general activities that are to be totaled and shown as management and general expenses in Exhibit B.

While for internal purposes it is possible to allocate management and general costs among the fund-raising and program service expense categories under a "full cost" accounting theory, the general nature of these activities requires that for external purposes they be reported separately. It is important to understand that this function is to be used to reflect only the indispensable stewardship and other costs needed to maintain the entity in order to deliver services—i.e., the costs included are identified on the basis of the nature of the expenses as discussed below and not whether they are "direct" or "indirect."

The extent to which particular salaries, travel, office and other expenses can be identified as clearly management and general expenses will vary widely among agencies. In a large national organization, executive direction, financial management, overall planning and the coordination of member unit activities may individually command the full time of several executives and separate clerical staffs. In smaller agencies, a single executive may devote part time to management functions, part to direct program activities and part to fund raising. The salary of this person will need to be charged, along with that of a secretary and other time-related expenses, such as travel, to each activity on the basis of the time devoted to each. Regardless, however, of size or structure, the *function* of management and general services exists in every organization.

Activities that agencies should classify as management and general services for reporting in Exhibit B include:

General board and committee meetings
Executive direction and corporate planning
General staff meetings
Office management
Corporate legal services
Personnel procurement
Purchasing and distribution of materials
Receptionist, switchboard, mail distribution, filing and other office services
Organization and procedure studies
Accounting, auditing, budgeting and external financial reporting
Internal financial and management reporting.

The above list is representative of common management and general activities. Other services—e.g., investment advice, executive training institutes—may have to be recognized by particular agencies as activities incurred in maintenance and direction of their total resources and reported as management and general. In some instances, on the other hand, some of the activities listed above can be reasonably and practically identified as part of another service—e.g., legal services secured specifically in connection with an agency's child adoption program and separately billed, or meetings of volunteer committees responsible for specific programs or fund-raising activities—and should be charged to the service benefited. Unless a reasonable, practical and verifiable basis exists for charging them directly to another service, however, activities of the type listed above should be accounted for as management and general. This includes, for instance, routine acknowledgment of and accounting for contributions and other income. However, the cost of maintaining detailed fund-raising records or of acknowledgements which include further appeals for funds should be charged to fund raising.

The costs of activities other than those listed above should be charged to the appropriate fund-raising or program service categories.

Internal financial and management, or administrative reporting—the last of the above-listed management and general activities—requires explanation and definition. Because of its close relation to public information, public relations and other types of public reporting by voluntary agencies, discussion of administrative reporting has been deferred to the section that deals with classification of all of an agency's informational activities.

Fund Raising

The usual voluntary health or welfare organization can no more leave to chance the financial support of its service programs than it can the management of whatever support it obtains. Fund-raising activity is vital and indispensable for almost every voluntary organization. In type and scope, fund-raising efforts of individual voluntary agencies range from nationwide appeals, employing virtually all of the persuasive techniques of major product advertising campaigns, to one or two appearances before budget committees of federated fund-raising organizations that have assumed the fund-raising responsibility for an agency.

Voluntary health and welfare agencies are expected to report as fund raising the expenses of all activities that constitute an appeal for financial support. By their own nature, fund-raising efforts may include a very wide range of activities. Illustrative of some types of fund-raising activities are:

1. Publicizing fund-raising campaigns and special events—e.g., by paid public relations counselors; by printed, radio and TV material; in meetings with potential contributors; through campaign "kick-off" dinners.
2. Conducting fund-raising campaigns, including services of fund-raising consultants; purchasing, preparing and maintaining mailing lists; recruiting and training volunteer solicitors and other campaign workers; solicitations in person or by mail; acquisition and distribution of seals and other enclosures with appeals for funds, of campaign kits, of coin containers and of other fund-raising materials.
3. Participation in local federated and Federal Service fund-raising campaigns including attendance at pre-campaign budget reviews.
4. Participation by employees of the agency benefited in fund-raising special events.
5. Solicitation of bequests, foundation grants and other special gifts—e.g., from corporations, from affluent individuals.
6. Clinics, workshops and other activities for improving fund-raising techniques.
7. Preparation and distribution of fund-raising manuals and instructions.

Object costs of the activities would include expenses of transmitting appeals to the public, such as postage and salaries (or portions of salaries) of personnel connected with the campaign engaged in addressing envelopes and maintenance of mailing lists.

Criteria for differentiating among and reporting activities that combine fund raising, educational and other kinds of information are examined in the second part of this chapter. Fund-raising services and materials purchased from affiliates should be charged to the Fund Raising function.

Fund-raising costs should generally be charged to the Current Unrestricted Fund. However, where fund-raising costs can be specifically identified with a special-purpose fund drive, such as a building-fund campaign, such costs should be charged to that Fund if legally appropriate, i.e., the restricted funds may be used to pay for the related fund-raising costs.

Federated fund-raising organizations (as described in Appendix 2) have a unique reporting problem because of their very nature. Therefore, they should use the reporting technique described in Appendix 2.

Deferral of Fund-Raising Expenses

Fund-raising efforts of one year, such as those made to obtain bequests or to compile a mailing list of prospective contributors, often result in contributions in future years. While the underlying accounting concept of matching revenues and expenses in the same period would theoretically justify deferral of fund-raising expenses in these circumstances, the uncertainty regarding the amount, if any, of such future contributions normally precludes deferral. Accordingly, fund-raising expenses should normally be expensed as incurred. However, if pledges or contributions restricted for future use are reflected as deferred contributions, related fund-raising costs, if specifically identifiable with the contributions, may also be deferred if there is positive evidence that the contributor(s) intended that such costs may be paid from the contributions. In addition, costs incurred in the acquisition of an inventory of literature and materials to be used in connection with a fund-raising drive to be conducted in a future period should be deferred to that period.

DISCLOSURE OF NATURE OF FUNCTIONAL EXPENSES

As has been discussed, the nature of program activities varies widely among voluntary health and welfare organizations, including those which utilize standard program categories. Accordingly, it is recommended that a brief description of each program and supporting service functional expense category be included in the operating statement (Exhibit B) or the notes to the financial statements. This will help to clarify the designations between program and supporting service expenses as well as provide the reader with a more complete understanding of the program service categories.

PAYMENTS TO AFFILIATED ORGANIZATIONS

This expense classification is used to report certain types of payments to organizations "affiliated with"—closely related to—a reporting agency.

Quota-support and dues payments (other than membership dues, as explained in the last part of this chapter) of local-national fund-raising campaign proceeds and possibly other types of payments (except for the purchase of goods or services which are treated as expenses in the usual manner) made by voluntary organizations to affiliates are to be identified as to purpose and reported in this classification. (See Exhibit B.) Payments by an affiliate to the national organization cannot normally be identified with any particular function and therefore are not functionally allocated on Exhibit C. However, footnote disclosure of the purposes for which such amounts are used can be made, if desired.

There may be cases where an agency would report certain types of payments to affiliates as a deduction from total support and revenue in the Statement of Revenue and Expenses and Changes in Fund Balances. Considerations in determining whether such treatment might be desirable include:

1. Contractual arrangements with the affiliated organization. Thus, for example, this criterion will have been met if the affiliate making the payment has a firm agreement with the organization that provides for a sharing of contributions raised by the affiliate on a fixed or determinable basis not subject to unilateral modification by either party.
2. Basis on which the funds are solicited and received from the public. This criterion expects that contributors are advised or are otherwise aware that funds contributed to the affiliate are shared with the other organization.

The discussion on awards and grants, later in this chapter, explains that an agency's expenses in support of specific programs may, under certain special conditions, be included in an appropriate program service classification, even though made to an affiliated organization. Payments to an affiliate for fund-raising expenses that the latter has incurred on behalf of the agency are to be reported as fund raising.

DIFFERENTIATING AMONG FUND-RAISING, PUBLIC EDUCATION AND OTHER INFORMATION MATERIALS AND ACTIVITIES

Among the most difficult of expense reporting problems confronting voluntary health and welfare organizations are those of accounting for materials and activities that may be described as "public education," "public information," "public relations," "publicity," and "fund raising." The gradation of meaning and connotations between these terms and the activities that they encompass suggest the complexity of the definition and expense reporting problem. Standards for distinguishing among these activities (and materials) and for uniform accounting and reporting of expenses that inextricably involve two or more of them are critical to fair financial reporting.

Criteria for Classifying Information Programs

As was earlier stated, functional reporting of an organization's expenses requires that they be grouped according to the activities for which they were incurred, and that expenses of particular activities be combined according to the program or purpose served. For example, the cost of a leaflet devoted exclusively to the nature and treatment of a disease, and distributed to the public primarily in doctors' offices or in hospitals, should be reported as public education. On the other hand, a folder on an agency's summer recreational activities for underprivileged children might be fully justifiable as expenses of the recreational program if distributed primarily among schools; distributed primarily to an audience of highly paid executives, however, it would normally have to be recognized as fund raising.

All circumstances surrounding certain activities and use of certain materials will need to be examined to determine their real purpose. Particular information pieces may be apparently educational in content, and yet be intended and used for no other purpose than to create an attitude of sympathy and receptivity toward a subsequent appeal for financial support—their real reason for distribution.

Public Education

For the purpose of uniform public reporting, public education is to be precisely defined and reported as a separate program function, as explained below.

Public education consists of information materials and activities:

1. Describing the symptoms of ill health, disease and physical or social disorders, or
2. Describing progress made in preventing or alleviating health or welfare problems, or
3. Describing actions to be taken by individuals or groups to prevent or alleviate personal or community health and welfare problems

and

Directed either to the general public or to special groups that may have a special need or special interest in the problem.

Public education is thus to be restricted to materials and activities that are problem- and not agency-oriented, and to efforts to tell individuals what *they* can or should do about a problem, not what an agency does or can do through available services.

Typical of materials and activities that should normally be accounted for as public education are the following:

School health lectures, posters, kits, etc.
Newspaper and magazine articles on health and welfare problems

Teacher-training programs and materials
Health problem check-lists, leaflets, models, etc.
Health or welfare handbooks and manuals for public distribution
Surveys for evaluation of education campaigns

Program Information for Participants and Leaders

Among the most important agency-oriented information programs of many agencies are those designed to interest particular groups in participating in or conducting one or another of an agency's primary service programs, such as day nurseries for children, recreation for senior citizens, etc. Such participating membership and leadership procurement activities or campaigns are often necessary program activities. They are to be accounted for, however, not as public education, but rather as expenses of the particular service or services to which they relate.

Fund-Raising Information

It is evident that even the most obviously educational publications, news releases and other informational activities of voluntary agencies may also have fund-raising value, if only as demonstrations of an agency's real service to the public and therefore entitlement to public support. The Fund-raising expense category can become very misleading, however, unless the information materials and activities which are included are restricted to those that are explicitly fund raising.

Administrative Reporting

Almost every voluntary health and welfare organization engages in some reporting and information programs that relate to the agency's services but that are not educational, program-supporting nor fund raising in terms of the above definitions. Representative of such reporting are printed annual reports, certain types of newsletters, and announcements of board and committee appointments and of research grants. The value of these reports and announcements in keeping an agency's name before the public, in drawing attention to its achievements and, therefore, in promoting public interest in and subsequent financial support of an agency is indisputable. It is equally clear that they also represent ways in which agencies discharge their proper and necessary obligation to account to the public for their stewardship of contributors' support.

Such general reporting may be referred to as "administrative reporting"—information materials and activities that:

1. Provide stewardship reporting on an agency in terms of service program and related achievements, and of professional, volunteer and financial resources used, or that
2. Provide general information directly related to their responsibilities to professional staff members, to volunteers working in and supervising an agency's service programs, and to others.

Illustrative of the first type are annual reports and meetings, newsletters and other bulletins that serve to keep an agency's constituency (including key community leaders and contributors) informed of its activities. House organs, bulletins and other pieces addressed primarily to professional staff members and to volunteers participating in an agency's service programs are examples of the second type.

The broad distribution of many forms of administrative reporting and their emphasis upon the activities of the sponsoring agency, as well as upon the health or welfare problems that are its concern, inevitably give them strong public relations and publicity value. Inescapably, administrative reporting also serves public information, institutional advertising and, therefore, fund-raising ends.

There is a real problem in classifying public information materials and activities that are neither explicitly and purely education—as previously defined—nor directly or specifically fund raising in character. It is no more practical to account separately for the fund-raising and administrative reporting components of a single annual report than it is, say, to segregate the costs of the packaging and advertising elements of an oatmeal box.

How, then, should the costs of information materials and activities that combine elements of public education, administrative reporting and potential future fund raising be accounted for in an agency's published financial statements. The logical basis for accounting for and reporting such activities is that they are general in purpose, supporting several of an agency's primary services (including fund raising)—and comparable, therefore, with the managerial, legal, accounting and other activities previously identified as management and general expenses. Thus, administrative reporting and other noneducational, nonprogram and non-fund-raising (as previously defined, in each instance) information materials and activities are to be accounted for in an agency's Exhibit B as management and general expenses.

Multiple-Purpose Information Materials and Activities

Very frequently, requests for financial support incorporate reports on an agency's activities or accomplishments. Often, such requests or appeals also contain information about health matters of benefit to the recipient.

In the development of the first edition of this book in 1964, the sponsoring organizations were highly concerned about the adverse impact on the credibility of nonprofit financial reporting resulting from several well-publicized scandals of the day. Accordingly, a standard was then adopted which called for allocation to fund raising of *all* multi-purpose information expenses, other than the incremental direct costs of separate educational pieces: This was called the "primary purpose" cost allocation concept. While this resulted in an overstatement of fund-raising expenses, the magnitude of error was rarely material. However, with changing economic and social conditions, particularly with the expanded use of computer-based direct mail combined educational and fund-raising programs, a number of organizations found strict application of this standard to cause concern about overstatements of fund-raising expenses.

In 1987, the American Institute of Certified Public Accountants (AICPA) issued Statement of Position 87-2, "Accounting for Joint Costs of Informational Materials and Activities of Not-For-Profit Organizations that Include a Fund-Raising Appeal." This document amended the AICPA's "Audits of Voluntary Health and Welfare Organizations" to clarify that a "primary purpose" approach to cost allocation was not in accordance with generally accepted accounting principles. Accordingly, *Standards* has been modified, to adopt SOP 87-2, as discussed in the following section.

Joint Mailings and Other Multiple-Part Information Efforts

The standards to be followed in allocation of joint costs of informational materials and activities that include a fund-raising appeal are as follows:

1. All joint costs of informational materials or activities that include a fund-raising appeal should be reported as fund-raising expense if it cannot be demonstrated that a program or management and general function has been conducted in conjunction with the appeal for funds. However, if it can be demonstrated that a bona fide program or management and general function has been conducted in conjunction with the appeal for funds, joint costs should be allocated between fund raising and the appropriate program or management and general function.
2. Demonstrating that a bona fide program or management and general function has been conducted in conjunction with an appeal for funds requires verifiable indications of the reasons for conducting the activity. Such indications include the content of the non-fund-raising portion of the activity; the audience targeted; the action, if any, requested of the recipients; and other corroborating evidence, such as written instruc-

tions to parties outside the organization that produce the activity, or documentation in minutes of the organization's board of the organization's reasons for the activity.

3. Most fund-raising appeals include descriptions of the causes for which the entities exist and the planned uses of the funds, to inform prospective donors about why funds are needed and what they will be used for. Unless such an appeal is designed to motivate its audience to action, other than providing financial support to the organization, all costs of the appeal should be charged to fund raising.
4. In order to accomplish their basic missions, some organizations educate the public and seek the involvement of the public in the attainment of their missions by telling people what they can or should do about particular issues. Those organizations should allocate joint costs to program activities if the informational materials or activities further those program goals.
5. Two examples of situations in which it may be appropriate to allocate such joint costs to program activities would be the following:
   a. A voluntary health and welfare organization describes the symptoms of a disease and the action an individual should take if those symptoms occur.
   b. An organization whose purpose is to raise public awareness alerts individuals to a social or community problem and urges their action in seeking changes.
6. Content of the message is an important factor, but content alone may not be a conclusive indication of the reason for the activity. For example, if an audience is selected principally because of the organization's perception of their need for or interest in the educational information, and not for their capacity to support the organization financially, any accompanying fund-raising appeal would appear to be incidental and the joint costs of the educational activity would not be required to be allocated. Conversely, if the audience is selected based on its presumed ability to provide financial support without consideration of its need for the educational information, the purpose would appear to be entirely fund raising, and all joint costs should be considered to be fund-raising costs regardless of any accompanying educational message.
7. All circumstances surrounding informational materials and activities that include a fund-raising appeal should be examined, and the criteria in paragraphs 1 through 6, above, should be applied together rather than separately.
8. Not-for-profit organizations incurring joint costs of informational materials and activities that include fund-raising appeals should disclose in their financial statements that such costs have been allocated, the

total amount allocated during the period, and the portion allocated to each functional expense category. The following illustrates such disclosure.

Note X. Allocation of Joint Costs

In 19XX, the organization incurred joint costs of ______for informational materials and activities that included fund-raising appeals. Of those costs, ______was allocated to fund-raising expense, ______was allocated to Program A expense, ______was allocated to Program B expense, and ______was allocated to management and general expense.

[Please see Appendix 8 for examples showing application of SOP 87-2.]

AWARDS AND GRANTS

Functional expense accounting and reporting by voluntary agencies require that special attention be given to awards and grants that agencies make to individuals and other organizations for a variety of purposes. The latter frequently include grants to individuals and to universities and other institutions unrelated to an agency. Many agencies also voluntarily make special research or other program grants to national affiliates, apart from and in addition to prescribed support quotas or percentages of local-national campaign proceeds they remit to the nationals.

The standard treatment of awards and grants requires that agencies account for them according to their ultimate purpose. Grants for research, for special studies, and for other projects that are natural extensions of one of an agency's service programs or consistent with a program purpose, should be reported as part of those program services expenses. In the case of payments to affiliated organizations, however, only payments that are voluntary on the part of an agency, subject to its own discretion and intended for specific service programs, may be reported as awards or grants in a functional category. (For treatment of other payments to affiliated organizations, see pages 50–51.)

Agencies that report awards and grants as program services expenses must disclose, parenthetically or otherwise, awards and grants for each program category made to affiliated organizations and the amount made to others. (See Exhibit C.)

Organizations that make grants to others should record grants as expenses and liabilities at the time recipients are entitled to them. That normally occurs when the grantee is notified; although some agencies recognize grant liabilities at the time of board approval. Some grants stipulate that payments are to be made over a period of several years. Grants payable in future periods, subject only to routine performance requirements by the grantee and not requiring subsequent review and approval for continuance of payment, should be recorded as expenses and liabilities when the grants are first made. However, if the grant instrument specifically states that the grantor reserves the right to discontinue grant payments, unpaid grants should not be recorded. Grants subject to such periodic renewal should be recorded as expenses and liabilities at the time of renewal with a disclosure of the remaining commitment in the notes to the financial statements. When practical, refunds and cancellations of prior-year grants should be offset against current grant expense and the amount disclosed.

OBJECT CATEGORIES IN STATEMENT OF FUNCTIONAL EXPENSES

Chapter III includes a general discussion of the purpose and format of Exhibit C, while a discussion of methods of allocating expenses among an agency's program and supporting service functions will be found in Appendix 1. The expenses to be included in each object classification listed on each line of Exhibit C are explained and illustrated below.

Agencies may use additional categories, may combine two or more categories into one, or may divide a category into two or more categories, if this is considered desirable for clear financial presentation, without obscuring necessary detail. The categories used should be consistent over time, and disclosure should be made of the nature of significant differences from the illustrated categories.

Salaries

Intended for: Salaries and wages earned by an agency's regular employees (full or part-time) and by temporary employees, including office temporaries, other than consultants and other persons engaged on an individual contract basis.

Illustrations:
Executive salaries
Professional staff salaries
Clerical salaries
Maintenance employees' wages
Bonus or incentive payments
Vacation and other compensated absences

Note: Individual agencies may subdivide this account—e.g., to show professional salaries separate from clerical and maintenance salaries and wages—as long as they show the totals of all salaries and wages opposite this caption on Exhibit C.

Employee Benefits

Intended for: Amounts paid and accrued by an agency under its own or other private employee health and retirement benefit plans, including voluntary employee termination or retirement payments outside a formal plan.

Illustrations:
Accident insurance premiums, or cost reimbursement
Medical and hospital plan premiums, or cost reimbursement
Pension or retirement plan contributions
Matching or other contributions to employee savings or similar plans
Other benefits (holiday gifts, use of recreational facilities, prepaid legal plan, etc.)

Payroll Taxes, Etc.

Intended for: Social Security taxes and compensation insurance premiums, payable by employers under Federal, state or local laws.

Illustrations:
F.I.C.A. payments (employer's share)
Unemployment insurance premiums
Worker's compensation insurance
Mandatory disability insurance premiums

Professional and Other Contract Service Fees

Intended for: Fees and expenses of professional practitioners and consultants who are not employees of the reporting agency and are engaged as independent contractors for specified services on a fee or other individual contract basis.

Illustrations:
Legal fees
Auditing and accounting fees and expenses
Contract payments to independent professional consultants
Fund-raising counsel fees
Actuarial fees
Data Processing Services (outside vendor)
Investment management fees (not commissions on transactions)
Contracted Software Development
Media Production Costs

Supplies

Intended for: Costs of materials, appliances and other supplies used by an agency.

Illustrations:
Medicines and drugs
Prosthetic appliances
Recreational and crafts materials
Food and beverages
Laundry, linen and housekeeping materials
Stationery, typing, accounting and other office materials
Paper, ink, film and duplicating materials

Telephone

Intended for: All telephone, telex and similar expenses.

Postage and Shipping

Intended for: Postage, parcel post, express mail, trucking and other delivery expenses, including shipping materials.

Occupancy

Intended for: All costs arising from an agency's occupancy and use of owned or leased land, buildings and offices. This excludes costs associated with housing but which are reported in other object categories—e.g., salaries, depreciation on buildings, insurance.

Illustrations:
Office rent
Electricity, heat and other utilities
Janitorial and other maintenance services under contract
Building and grounds maintenance supplies

Interest Expense

Intended for: Interest incurred on mortgage notes, capitalized equipment leases, and other short- or long-term debt.

Rental and Maintenance of Equipment

Intended for: Cost of renting and maintaining equipment (such as electronic data processing units, typewriters, calculators, dictaphones), including program and other equipment. The rental and maintenance of automotive vehicles should be included in travel/transportation.

Printing and Publications

Intended for: Costs of printing, commercial artists and suppliers for plates, advertising, art work, proofs, photographs and other costs of house organs, leaflets, films and other information materials, including the cost of purchased publications, technical journals, books, pamphlets and monographs.

Travel and Transportation

Intended for: Expenses of travel and transportation for staff and volunteers of the reporting agency.

Illustrations:
Transportation fees, mileage allowances, hotel, meals and incidental expenses
Local bus and taxicab fares
Automobile expenses of operating agency-owned or leased vehicles used for programs or general purposes, except insurance
Allowances for use of employees' or volunteers' automobiles on business for agency

Conferences, Conventions and Meetings

Intended for: Expenses of conducting or attending meetings related to an agency's activities, other than travel costs which should be included in the preceding category.

Illustrations:
Meeting space and equipment rentals
Meeting program, notices, badges and related printing costs
Cost of organized meals
Speakers' honorariums and expenses
Conference and convention registration fees for agency staff participants

Specific Assistance to Individuals

Intended for: The cost to the reporting agency of assistance or services for a particular client or patient, including assistance rendered by others at the expense of the reporting agency.

Illustrations:
Medical, dental and hospital fees and charges
Children's board
Homemaker services
Client and patient travel
Food, shelter and clothing

Individual camperships

Note: This category is also designed to include materials and appliances furnished by the reporting agency when purchased for or identifiable with a particular client or patient.

Membership Dues

Intended for: Amounts paid or payable for bona fide membership in other organizations which provide, in return, benefits such as regular services, publications, materials, etc.

Note: This category covers payments of the type that are to be reported as other revenue by receiving health and welfare organizations. For example, national organizations include such amounts received in assessments and dues from local member units. (See Chapter IV.) Payments that do not procure, for the paying agency, general membership benefits, as described in Chapter IV, should be reported as contributions as described in the sections on awards and grants and payments to affiliated organizations earlier in this chapter.

Awards and Grants

Intended for: Amount paid or committed to individuals or organizations for support of research, fellowship, scholarship and other health or welfare programs. Amounts paid to affiliated organizations should be reported separately from amounts paid to others. (See Exhibit C.)

Illustrations:

Grants to research institutions

Graduate fellowships

Trainee scholarships

Allowances for travel and equipment under particular awards or grants

Contributions or grants which are formula-based or prescribed payments by an agency in support of an affiliate should not be shown opposite this caption (See the section on payments to affiliated organizations in this chapter.)

Insurance

Intended for: All costs of insurance except employee benefits or other payroll-related insurance (worker's compensation, disability, unemployment). Should include property insurance, general liability, professional liability (—e.g., malpractice), fidelity bonds, directors' and officers' liability, automobile and other vehicles, meeting cancellation, business interruption insurance. (Should not include insurance provided to beneficiaries of an agency's programs—included with Specific Assistance to Individuals.)

Other Expenses

Intended for: All expenses not reportable in another object classification.

Depreciation or Amortization

Intended for: Allocation of the cost, or other carrying value, of physical assets over their estimated useful lives. Provision for depreciation or amortization is an accounting process intended to spread the cost of such assets over the period of time their use benefits the program or supporting activities of the agency; it should not be viewed as a means of funding their replacement.

Illustrations:
Depreciation—equipment
Amortization—leasehold improvements and capital leases
Depreciation—automotive equipment
Depreciation—buildings

CHAPTER VI

REPORTING OF ASSETS, LIABILITIES AND FUND BALANCES

Annual reporting to the public is incomplete if confined to an agency's operating statements, Exhibits B and C in Chapter VIII. The public is also entitled to know the nature and carrying values of all significant assets an agency owns and of debts it owes, and to see that the agency recognizes necessary distinctions between assets, liabilities and Fund balances that must be accounted for separately, as discussed in Chapter II. To present this further evidence of their stewardship of the public's support, voluntary health and welfare organizations should include in their annual published financial statements a Balance Sheet conforming in content and format, to the extent appropriate for each organization, to Exhibit A in Chapter VIII.

PRESENTATION OF FUNDS

The most conspicuous difference between Exhibit A and the balance sheets with which laymen are generally familiar is that Exhibit A presents not one, but four separate balance sheets—one for each of the agency's Funds: one for the Current Unrestricted Fund, one for the Current Restricted Fund, one for the Land, Building and Equipment Fund and one for the Endowment Fund. Each Fund includes assets of the Fund and the Fund balance or balances and may include one or more liability and deferred support or revenue accounts. Segregation, in a Balance Sheet, of at least the fund balances of each Fund is essential to show the extent to which an agency has honored restrictions attached to gifts by particular donors—e.g., to show that contributions to an Endowment Fund have been accounted for separately and not included in accounts of funds available for unrestricted purposes. In addition, segregation of assets and liabilities may be desirable in circumstances when the assets of separate Funds are not interchangeable.

Material amounts of assets held in trust for the benefit of an agency by an outside trustee should be disclosed by the agency. However, since such funds are not under the control of the benefited agency, they generally should not be included in its Balance Sheet; the facts of the trust arrangement, to the extent they are ascertainable, should be disclosed in a note accompanying the agency's financial statements.

THE CONTENT AND PRESENTATION OF INDIVIDUAL BALANCE SHEET ACCOUNTS

The reader's understanding of financial statements published by similar organizations will be improved by agencies' adherence to uniform terminology. To the extent possible, voluntary health and welfare agencies should conform their Balance Sheet account titles and content to those presented in Exhibit A and described below. Neither Exhibit A nor the following discussions purport, however, to be all-inclusive; individual agencies should supplement or expand the accounts described here for adequate disclosure of particular assets or liabilities. On the other hand, some accounts may not be required. Agencies may select those accounts for reporting that reflect their particular assets, liabilities and Fund balances. An account may be combined with another account of a similar type if the amount in one of the accounts alone is insignificant.

Cash

Assets are normally listed in a balance sheet with the most liquid items shown first. Thus cash, whose liquidity is usually absolute, should be the first caption in a Balance Sheet. This item should include all cash actually held by an agency. Cash on deposit in checking accounts, deposits in transit, change funds and petty cash funds held for operating purposes may properly be combined. Cash deposited in interest-bearing accounts such as N.O.W. accounts or savings accounts (including money market accounts) should be disclosed on the statement or in a footnote.

An item should not be recorded as cash until the money is actually received by an agency. It is improper, for example, to show receivables as cash prior to the date of their actual collection.

Short-Term Investments

Short-term investments appear next after cash because of their liquidity. They represent temporary investments of cash not immediately required. Examples are United States Treasury bills, certificates of deposit, bankers acceptances, repurchase agreements, and commercial paper. They are usually quickly convertible into cash, and their maturities may range anywhere from a few days to a year. It should be recognized, however, that the distinction between short-term and noncurrent investments is not the nature of the investment but rather the intention of the organization with regard to the timing of its conversion into cash.

Accounts Receivable

An asset group on the balance sheet of many agencies will be accounts receivable of one form or another. Accounts receivable frequently result from an agency's program services. They may also arise through operation of revenue-producing activities, such as sales of materials or publications. Reimbursements due from affiliates, claims against vendors and even advances to staff members are other receivables that may be sufficiently important to require separate disclosure in an agency's Balance Sheet.

For consistency with accrual accounting as the recognized basis for public financial reporting by voluntary health and welfare agencies, uncollected accounts receivable of an agency as of its fiscal year-end should be shown in its Balance Sheet. Accounts receivable from all sources other than contributors (pledges—see next section) are included in accounts receivable. An agency should also show in the Balance Sheet, or in a footnote, the nature and amounts of significant individual classes of accounts receivable included in the total shown—e.g., clients or customers, government agencies, etc. In addition, significant receivables from related parties such as employees, volunteers, affiliated organizations, etc., should be presented separately or otherwise disclosed.

Accounts receivable should be analyzed, at least for annual Balance Sheet reporting, as to the likelihood of their being collected in full. Any allowance for uncollectible accounts that may be considered necessary, on the basis of the analysis, should be shown as a deduction from the related receivable in the Balance Sheet. The change in the allowance for the year (whether an increase or decrease) is included in the appropriate expense category for the year reported in Exhibit B.

Pledges Receivable

A frequently raised question about financial reporting to the public is related to the problems of accounting for pledges receivable. Some argue that including these is impractical because it requires highly questionable estimates as to the amounts that may be collected, and because voluntary agencies are in no position, presumably, to enforce collection of pledges.

For many voluntary health and welfare agencies, however, contributions by way of pledges are too important to be overlooked. For example, many federated fund-raising organizations encourage contributors to make pledges rather than cash contributions and to pay them by regular payroll deductions or installment payments. Building-fund drives or other campaigns of voluntary agencies also often receive large grants that are payable in installments. Nor can an agency ignore a pledge from a regular contributor simply because payment is deferred until the beginning of the next year. In other words, an agency has an obligation to report, in its financial statements, significant pledges that are reasonably certain to be collected.

If total omission of significant pledges from an agency's financial statements is indefensible, mechanical reporting of all pledges received by an agency is no more acceptable. Before pledges may properly be included in an agency's support and revenue for a year and in its year-end Balance Sheet, they must be evaluated as to the likelihood of payment.

With experience and a systematic approach, the evaluating process can become reasonably accurate. Agencies can usually identify certain pledges as unlikely ever to be paid, others as quite reliable. One practical way to evaluate pledges still unpaid is to "age" them—to group them according to the time which has passed since they were to have been paid. Groups might be established for those not yet due, those up to thirty days old, thirty to sixty days old, sixty to ninety days old, etc. With experience, a reasonable factor usually can be developed for the percentage of each group that probably will be collected. Use of the aging technique requires only that an agency keep records of payments on pledges to which it can refer as a basis for estimating the probable yield of future pledges of different ages. Another way to evaluate pledges, which might be used by United Ways and federated fund-raising organizations that receive pledges payable through payroll deduction, is to analyze historical trends of collection by company, industry, or employee group.

In Exhibit B, amounts pledged are reported as public support in the year the support is available for use after deducting allowances for amounts that may prove uncollectible. The amounts to be shown as pledges receivable in Exhibit A, on the other hand, are the totals, again after allowing for estimated uncollectible amounts, of all pledges unpaid at the balance sheet date. These include not only pledges received in the current year, but also amounts receivable from years prior to the current year. The purely voluntary character of pledges, in most instances, makes it necessary that they be presented separately from other receivables.

Such reporting of pledges in an agency's balance sheet clearly requires that an agency, at least annually, re-evaluate its prior years' receivables with particular care and possibly write off some, and increase allowances for uncollectibility with respect to others. Any resulting adjustments should be added to or deducted from the respective public support category in an agency's current year Exhibit B. If uncollected pledges are carefully evaluated and included in each year's Balance Sheet at realistic values, subsequent years' adjustments and write-offs should not significantly affect the amounts reported as current public support each year.

Donors will sometimes make a pledge in one year which is intended to be paid in a subsequent year. Until the year of intended payment and use, these pledges do not fully belong to an agency. If an agency had received payments against pledges that had been specified for use in a future year, and had to go out of business before the year in question, it might be obliged to refund the amounts collected. Until the year for which they are available for use, such pledges should be reported as deferred income (support and revenue designated for future periods) in its year-end Balance Sheet. The governing factor is the donor's intent. If a donor specifically indicates that his/her contribution is for use in a particular year, obviously that is the intent. However, where a pledge is payable in installments, unless the donor specifies otherwise, the contribution should be included in support in the years the installments become due. If the donor does not specify a period of intended payment, the pledge should be assumed to be for current support.

Inventory

The inventory category refers to materials and goods purchased or manufactured by or donated to an organization and held to be sold, either to affiliated or other agencies or to the public, or to be used in operations in some future period. These items are real assets at the date of the Balance Sheet, because they represent something of value, have a specific price, are on hand and have not yet been distributed or used. If they were not on hand, the agency would have to purchase them. As to the future, they represent either expenses which will be applied to future operations or items for sale for which an agency will later collect cash. The range of items for possible reporting in this asset classification may include bulletins and literature on hand that can be used in the future—e.g., in fund-raising activities—food to be used in a summer camp, supplies for camping activities, insignia, printed lesson material, medicines and materials to be distributed to welfare recipients or to other agencies in connection with agency programs. They should be valued and presented in an agency's Balance Sheet, however, only if they can be sold, or to the extent that they can be expected to contribute to some future program of the agency. Items which have been donated may be included in this caption, if they meet the above requirement, to the extent of the values at which they have been recorded as contributions, as discussed below.

Inventory should be recorded on the Balance Sheet at the lower of: (1) actual cost, (2) the amount for which they are to be sold in the case of items for sale, or (3) in the case of material to be used in future operations, the value they still have for the organization's purposes.

Written-off Materials

It sometimes becomes necessary to make adjustments in amounts of inventory because items held have lost their value. This may occur because of spoilage or damage or because of obsolescence resulting from a change in program. Materials for fund-raising purposes are such an example. If these materials are procured in advance for a campaign and are being held for distribution at the time of the statement, they should be shown as inventory. If they are dated or otherwise unusable for subsequent campaigns, however, they should not be included in inventory. Deteriorated or unusable materials should be written off by charging the cost to the function for which they were originally acquired.

Prepaid Expenses and Deferred Charges

To provide comparable and consistent reporting of support, revenue and expenses, it may be necessary to make accounting adjustments to carry forward, or defer to the following year, expense prepayments of a material amount—e.g., insurance—applicable to future years, or expenses properly to be related to a future year's activities, such as advance expenses for the following year's fund-raising campaign. These items are to be carried in the Balance Sheet until the period for which they are proper expenses.

Only those fund-raising expenses specifically identifiable with fund-raising efforts to be undertaken in future years may be deferred. In most cases, no portion of expenses related to current efforts may be deferred, even though some of the resulting contributions may not be received until future years. An exception to this rule would apply to federated fund-raising organizations, which may defer fund-raising expenses until the year of distribution of the proceeds from a campaign (see discussion of this point on pp. 105–106).

Non-Current Investments

This investment caption is used to report assets intended to be held for periods of time longer than a year for income-producing purposes. As contrasted with short-term, the purpose of non-current investments is not to seek early recovery of principal, but to obtain continuing investment income and/or capital appreciation.

Exhibit A reflects two groups of long-term investments. The first is board-designated, non-current investments of the Current Unrestricted Fund, which the governing board may use at its own discretion. The second, investments of the Endowment Fund, is restricted by donors and subject to the terms of the gifts and/or legacies.

Non-current investments might consist of government bonds, corporate stocks and bonds or even real estate. Note that this caption can also include investments maturing in a short time if the intention is to reinvest the proceeds. Where the amounts of investments are significant, the types of assets held for this purpose should be specified. It is desirable, for example, to separate readily marketable securities from less readily marketable investments such as real estate.

An agency may own such a large percentage of the stock of one company that the company is effectively controlled by the agency, and accounting on the equity method or full consolidation is appropriate.

Investments purchased by voluntary health and welfare organizations should be initially recorded at cost, which includes brokerage, taxes and other charges directly applicable to the purchase. Securities donated to the organization should be recorded at their fair market value at the date of the gift (best measured by the net proceeds if sold shortly after receipt). If the market value of the investment portfolio is below the recorded value, it may be necessary to reduce the carrying value of the portfolio to market, or to provide an allowance for decline in market value. If it can be reasonably expected that the the asset value has been permanently impaired and, therefore, that the organization will suffer a loss on disposition of the investment, provision should be made during the period in which the decline in value occurred.

As an alternative, organizations may elect to report investments on a market value basis in their financial statements. If investments are carried at market, the change (whether positive or negative) in unrealized appreciation (or depreciation) should be included in revenue of the appropriate Fund in the Statement of Revenue and Expenses and Changes in Fund Balances.

The basis of carrying investments should be the same in all Funds and should be clearly disclosed in the financial statements. Where investments are carried at cost, the total market value of investments at the date of the statements should be shown parenthetically or set forth in the notes to the financial statements. (For a discussion of investment pools, see Chapter IV and Appendix 3.)

Fixed Assets and Depreciation

The stewardship and reporting responsibility of voluntary agencies extends to land, buildings and equipment (whether purchased, donated, or financed by contributors), no less than to cash and other assets. Contributors whose donations have been used to acquire property are entitled to know what their dollars have bought, and readers of an agency's financial statements are entitled to see in its Balance Sheet all important assets for which its management is responsible.

Voluntary agencies usually acquire items of property and equipment either by purchase or by gift. Fixed assets may be held by the organization for use, for investment, or for sale.

Inextricably involved with fixed assets is the question of depreciation of these assets. The following sections describe accounting for the acquisition, depreciation and replacement of fixed assets by voluntary health and welfare organizations.

1. Agencies should account for and report separately fixed assets held for investment or sale, and those held for use. Assets held for investment or sale should be included in the current or the Endowment Fund, as appropriate to any donor restrictions on the property. If amounts of such assets are significant, they should be separately disclosed. Amounts reported on the Balance Sheet should be as discussed above under non-current investments.

   A separate Land, Building and Equipment Fund should be maintained in the agency's accounting records to record transactions relating to assets, depreciation, mortgages, other liabilities, and Fund balances involving fixed assets held for use by an organization, and for contributions restricted by donors for the acquisition or construction of fixed assets for use. "Held for use" are the key words. No other assets (fixed or otherwise) or liabilities should be carried in this Fund unless they relate to this purpose. Such a Fund is shown separately both on the Statement of Revenue and Expenses and Changes in Fund Balances (Exhibit B) and the Balance Sheet (Exhibit A). Since the sources of the funds used to acquire fixed assets often are a combination of unrestricted resources and resources restricted for the purchase of fixed assets, it may not be clear whether proceeds from later sale of assets purchased with restricted funds continue to bear the original donor restrictions. Resolution of this issue is a legal matter.
2. An agency's Land, Building and Equipment Fund Balance Sheet, or the notes thereto, should normally show separate totals for land, for buildings (and equipment built into them) and for its furniture, furnishings and office equipment which are owned, or are rented under leases which are capital leases. Even so-called "fixed" assets exhibit wide differences in real value; land has lasting value, while automobiles, for instance, become uneconomical to operate in a relatively short time. Segregation of an agency's fixed asset values into types, as indicated above, assists readers of its Balance Sheet to understand the relative significance of values shown for different classes of property. The particular assets owned by a given agency may call either for a classification different from that shown in Exhibit A—e.g., canoes that represent a major equipment category of an agency camp—or for subdivision of one of the above classifications. The objective sought in classifying an agency's fixed assets should be to group assets similar in nature.

3. Purchased fixed assets should be recorded at actual cost and donated assets at their fair market value at the date of the gift. Actual cost may include an agent's fees, acquisition costs, freight, installation, and sales taxes, and other costs incurred in addition to the asset cost. In the absence of adequate cost records, appraisals of historical cost or market value at date of the gift are acceptable for initial valuation for financial reporting purposes. If assets are constructed for the organization, and if they are financed with borrowed money, it may be necessary to capitalize interest incurred during construction on the borrowing as part of the cost of the assets and disclose in the notes the policy and the amount of interest capitalized.
4. Depreciation of fixed assets held for use should be included as an element of expenses in the Statement of Functional Expenses, and also in the Statement of Revenue and Expenses and Changes in Fund Balances in the Land, Building and Equipment Fund. Fixed assets should be reported net on the balance sheet with accumulated depreciation disclosed on the statement or in a footnote.
5. An agency that desires to set aside or appropriate funds for self-financing of fixed asset replacement may do so by board action. It should report the appropriation under the "designated by the governing board" classification in the Current Unrestricted Fund balance of the Balance Sheet. (See also the discussion of reserves and appropriations in Chapter II.)
6. Methods of valuing fixed assets, depreciable lives, and methods of computing depreciation should be disclosed.

The principle that voluntary agencies report the values of the fixed assets they own in their Balance Sheets raises a number of practical accounting questions. What are the "fixed assets"? How far are voluntary agencies expected to go in attempting to inventory, set up detailed records for, and value items of equipment? Are voluntary agencies expected to show in their own balance sheets land and buildings that they occupy and use but that are owned by another organization (as in the case, for instance, with many church-sponsored agencies)? On what basis are agencies expected to value assets acquired over a period of years for which no cost records are available? How are donated items of property and equipment to be valued? Although these last two questions have been previously answered to some extent, more attention will be given to them in the following discussion.

Voluntary agencies are not required to show in their own Balance Sheet any values for land, buildings and equipment they occupy and use but which are owned by another organization. Agencies so favored should disclose the facts, however, in a note to their financial statements—e.g.: "The accompanying financial statements do not reflect the value of the land and buildings occupied by the agency, as these are recorded in the name of the Bishop of the Diocese of ___________." However, as was discussed in Chapter IV, the rental value of contributed space should be reported both as a contribution and as an expense to reflect occupancy.

On the other hand, if an agency occupies real property owned by, for example, a governmental unit, and the government has agreed that the agency shall have use of the property for an indefinite period, the agency may choose to include the property on its Balance Sheet. Similarly, an agency may have acquired fixed assets with money from a grant in which the grantor retains a reversionary interest in the property at the end of the grant period. In many such situations, the grantor, in fact, typically lets the agency retain the property. Such property may also be included on the agency's Balance Sheet. In both situations, full disclosure of the circumstances surrounding the property should be made.

Small items of office equipment, minor furnishings, hand tools and the like, on the other hand, are generally too numerous and of too little individual value to warrant the effort to inventory and value them. An arbitrary minimum value (except for groups of items substantial in amount) might be established below which individual items or groups of items would not be capitalized, but would be reported as expenses when acquired. This minimum value will vary based on the size of the agency.

Donated Land, Buildings and Equipment

As indicated, the standards discussed previously for accounting for land, buildings and equipment apply to donated as well as to purchased property. It is recognized, nonetheless, that agencies occasionally receive donations of furnishings, furniture and other items for which they have little need or which are of much finer quality than they could normally afford. If the agency intends to dispose of the items, they should be recorded in the unrestricted fund at their fair value at the date of the gift. If the agency intends to use the items, or if the donor has restricted the gift in such a way that the organization cannot dispose of it, then the value should be a figure that realistically suits the circumstances. For example, an unusually expensive donation would be adjusted to its "utility" value to the organization. It may be necessary to explain the accounting treatment in a note to the agency's financial statements, depending on materiality.

Accounts Payable and Accrued Expenses

While this account will normally appear in the Current Unrestricted Fund, it may also appear in other Funds. Two types of "unpaid" items need to be recognized, at least in an agency's year-end accounting. The first consists of "bills," invoices for individual purchases or statements summarizing a month's transactions—e.g., cleaning services, electricity, telephone charges. These are referred to as "accounts payable." The second group encompasses expenses that accumulate, or accrue, to some extent automatically, with the passage of time. Rent, salaries, (and related fringe benefits such as payroll taxes and vacation pay), property taxes and mortgage interest payments are examples. "Accrued expenses" is the term used to describe liabilities of this type. Other liabilities requiring recognition, if they exist, in an agency's balance sheet may include such debts as bank loans or loans from an affiliated organization, and amounts due under capital leases. Payables would also include grants payable to others as discussed on pp. 57–58.

Support and Revenue Designated for Future Periods

This is a deferred revenue caption under which an agency should group, with details appropriate to the magnitude and types of support or revenue involved, items such as contributions (including contributions to capital campaigns), governmental fees or grants, foundation grants, membership dues, other fees and support that contributors or grantors have designated as payable for or applicable to a future year either by terms of the gift, whether it be in the form of cash or pledge, or by terms of contract, type of solicitation, or other arrangement. Examples are deferral of pledged contributions and other support, and of amounts of grants definitely committed for or applicable to future years. It should not be used to accumulate "reserves" or contingency appropriations, which would impair comparability of agencies' balance sheets and be misleading to contributors.

The unspent portion of gifts or other revenue restricted by donors and grantors for specific purposes, but without a restriction as to time period of use, should not be recorded as deferred revenue. All such revenue should be recorded as revenue when the organization is entitled to receive payment. The unspent portion will then be included in the Fund balance of the Current Restricted Fund.

Interfund Receivables and Payables

Interfund accounts will be required if an agency makes interfund loans. Other interfund accounts may arise from the common and acceptable practice of initially recording transactions, affecting any of an agency's Funds, in the Current Unrestricted Fund. Materials chargeable to a Fund restricted to support of research, for instance, might be paid for from a general bank account (maintained for more than one Fund) and be charged, initially, to an account of the Current Unrestricted Fund. Afterwards, an entry would be made in the latter Fund crediting the account and charging the expenses to the appropriate account for research in the Current Restricted Fund.

For annual public reporting purposes, it is desirable that such interfund accounts be eliminated as far as practicable—i.e., as indicated in the above illustration—by a bookkeeping entry or, where separate bank accounts are maintained for each Fund, by an actual cash transfer restoring the amount paid for the supplies to the current Unrestricted Fund cash balance and reducing the Research Fund cash. The advantage gained in eliminating interfund accounts is that individual Fund balance sheets will then show the actual cash balances available to meet their respective external liabilities and future expenses.

If it becomes evident that contemplated sources of funds for repayment of interfund receivables will not be available in the foreseeable future, such loans should be considered permanent, and should be recorded as transfers of funds, by charging the lending funds, crediting the borrowing funds, and eliminating the interfund balances.

There may be legal prohibitions against lending such funds and against recording such transfers. If so, appropriate disclosure should be made. Material interfund borrowings should be disclosed when restricted funds have been loaned or when the liquidity of either fund is in question.

When the columnar format (Exhibit A) is used, it is preferable to present interfund balances entirely on one line in the asset section, adding across to zero (the fund which shows the payable will report it as a negative number) to avoid overstating the aggregate assets and liabilities of the entity as a whole.

Other Assets and Liabilities

Voluntary health and welfare organizations vary so widely in size, programs and financing that it is impractical to attempt to devise an all-inclusive classification of balance sheet accounts for them. Only the major classes of assets and liabilities with which most voluntary agencies will have to deal in seeking to achieve uniform public financial reporting have been considered here. Circumstances of individual agencies may, for example, require accounting for mortgage obligations, long-term notes payable or other assets and liabilities substantially identical with those of commercial entities.

CLASSIFIED BALANCE SHEET

Many organizations have only unrestricted funds. Those organizations may wish to classify their assets as current, fixed, or other long-term assets and their liabilities as current or long-term. To be classified as "current," the assets generally should be realizable and the liabilities payable within a normal operating cycle. However, if there is no normal operating cycle or the operating cycle is less than one year, all assets expected to be converted to cash or other liquid resources within one year, and all liabilities to be liquidated within one year, should be classified as current.

Other organizations have both unrestricted and restricted funds. Frequently, the fund classifications themselves adequately disclose the current and long-term nature of the assets and liabilities. If not, a classified balance sheet may be presented.

APPROPRIATIONS—BOARD-DESIGNATED FUNDS

Some nonprofit organizations have, on occasion, created general "reserves" or made general appropriations from balances of unrestricted funds. In some instances, funds were segregated to provide for specific contingencies or other future needs, the financial requirements of which were at the moment indeterminate. Such reserves, appropriations or contingencies should not be included as liabilities, or as separate funds on an agency's balance sheet. However, the procedure that follows does provide an acceptable method for recording provisions for ascertainable future needs.

Where a board wishes to indicate in the Current Unrestricted Fund balance sheet that it intends to use some portion of the Fund balance in a future period for a particular purpose, it may do so by designating part of the Fund balance. Such designations should be documented in the board minutes. For example, if the board wishes to designate $115,200 for future research purposes, the agency would report the designation within the Fund balance section as follows:

Designated by the governing board for—
Research purposes $115,200
(This presentation can be seen in Exhibit A.)

It should be noted that this designation does not result in a charge reflected in Exhibit B. Rather, all that has happened is that the board has segregated a portion of its Current Unrestricted Fund balance to indicate its intention to spend these monies in a certain way. During a future period, when the amounts for research are actually expended, they will be included in the expenses of the Current Unrestricted Fund in Exhibit B. The agency would then reverse its designation in the Fund balance section.

Usually it would not be necessary to show the details of all changes during the year in the amounts designated for specific purposes by the board on the balance sheet. Disclosure of the year-end balances in the Balance Sheet would normally be sufficient. If, on the other hand, the board wished to disclose the details, it could do so in the notes to the financial statements or in a separate statement of changes in fund balances.

The undesignated balance should not be reported to be in deficit position as the result of designations which exceed the total available unrestricted fund balance.

FUND BALANCES

The presentation of the balances of individual Funds in an agency's Balance Sheet should conform to the nomenclature illustrated in Exhibit A and to the sub-classification standards discussed in Chapter II.

CHAPTER VII

COMBINING FINANCIAL STATEMENTS OF CLOSELY RELATED ORGANIZATIONS

This chapter covers both combined and combining financial statements. Combined financial statements present only the total combined "entity," whereas combining financial statements present separately some or all of the individual entities included. Wherever the term "combined" is used, it also covers combining financial statements, if such statements are preferred.

Situations exist in which voluntary health and welfare organizations are so closely related that they may reasonably be regarded as a single entity, and their financial reports should be combined in a single set of statements. For instance, a national organization that permits solicitation of contributions in its name by local affiliates may be expected to account for all the programs served by the contributor's dollar—nationally as well as locally—in a single set of financial statements. The same may be said of a local agency that permits an auxiliary or other volunteer group to appeal for financial support on its behalf. In such instances, only the ultimate recipient, or central organization, may be in a position to render a combined report of all program and supporting service uses to which contributions to any of the related agencies have been applied.

Other circumstances, apart from a central organization's permitting solicitation of support in its name by affiliated organizations, may call for combined financial reporting for a group of related agencies. If major program services—e.g., research, health education, direct services to individuals—or fund-raising activities of one organization are substantially financed by its affiliates, or when local fund raising is substantially financed by a national organization, combined financial statements for the organization and its affiliates may be indispensable for accounting to contributors to the affiliates for an important part of their contributions. If a central organization effectively has final control over the funds of one or more related organizations so as to be able to direct their use and accounting, or if the related organizations have no significant programs apart from financial support of the central organization, combined financial reporting for the central organization and its related agencies or other groups will usually be essential for complete and meaningful financial disclosure.

STANDARDS FOR THE COMBINING OF FINANCIAL STATEMENTS

Combined financial statements may provide better information than separate statements. However, the state of the art in this area is in flux. The AICPA industry audit guide, "Audits of Voluntary Health and Welfare Organizations," indicates that the question "revolves around the functions performed by the organizations" and "the extent to which their operations and finances are interlocked."

The FASB is studying the issue of what constitutes the reporting entity and final accounting standards must await the conclusion of that effort.

Voluntary health and welfare organizations should adopt combined reporting when it is helpful in achieving comprehensive accounting to the public for activities of units effectively controlled—e.g., for a local agency and supporting auxiliaries, for a state organization and its local chapters.

SOP 78-10 states that: "for a reporting organization that controls another organization having a compatible purpose, it is presumed that combined financial statements are more meaningful than separate statements and are usually necessary for a fair presentation in conformity with generally accepted accounting principles. Control means the direct or indirect ability to determine the direction of the management and policies through ownership, by contract, or otherwise."

Combined financial statements are preferable for informative presentation of certain interrelated organizations. Combined financial statements should be presented if (1) control exists, as defined above, and (2) any of the following circumstances exist:

a. Separate entities solicit funds in the name of and with the expressed or implicit approval of the reporting organization, and substantially all of the funds solicited are intended by the contributor, or are otherwise required to be transferred to the reporting organization, or used at its discretion or direction.
b. A reporting organization transfers some of its resources to another separate entity whose resources are held for the benefit of the reporting organization.
c. A reporting organization assigns functions to a controlled entity whose funding is primarily derived from sources other than public contributions, such as a research entity supported by government grants.

For annual reporting pursuant to these standards, a voluntary health and welfare organization should present a single set of combined financial statements for itself, and for all of its affiliated organizations or groups to which any one of the foregoing criteria applies. They should be understood as applicable both to local and to national organizations, and to unincorporated auxiliaries, guilds, circles, committees and other organized groups associated with a health or welfare organization, as well as to incorporated organizations.

Legally unrestricted resources held by organizations related to the reporting organization may be effectively restricted with respect to the reporting organization. In combined financial statements that include both the related organization and the reporting organization, it may be appropriate to present all resources of the related organization, both unrestricted and restricted, as restricted resources.

A national or international organization may have state or local chapters with varying degrees of autonomy. Affiliated organizations may be separate corporate entities or unincorporated boards, committees, or chapters. A national or "parent" organization with loosely affiliated local organizations whose resources are principally derived and expended locally, normally would not combine the local organizations' financial statements with its own. Some of the characteristics of a loose affiliation are:

1. Locally determined program activities
2. Financial independence of the local organization
3. Control of its assets by the local organization

See section below "Combined Financial Statements: A Case Study."

Disclosure of Basis of Financial Statement Combination

The basis for combining financial statements should be disclosed in the notes to the financial statements, including the interrelationship of the combined organizations, and a description of the entities.

If affiliated organizations are not combined because they do not meet the above combining criteria, the existence of the affiliates and their relationships to the reporting organizations should be disclosed.

Financial reporting that purports to present the combined financial statements of a group of related organizations may fairly be assumed, in the absence of qualifying explanations, to include all affiliates of the reporting organization. When such statements omit any organizations closely related to the reporting organization, the basis for the omission should be clearly described in the headings of the statements or in a note accompanying them.

CONFORMING SUBORDINATE UNIT ACCOUNTING TO COMBINED FINANCIAL REPORTING

In combining financial statements of related organizations, the final step is the addition of all major report classifications of the related organizations to obtain totals for the entire group. If the total in each resulting accounting classification is to conform to the respective definition in this report, the individual accounts of the organizations being combined must be maintained in conformity with the definitions in *Standards*. In addition, central and affiliated organizations must maintain reciprocal accounts for transactions with each other—e.g., collected through local member units and paid to national organization on the books of a national organization—campaign proceeds on the books of a local. This will permit elimination of intragroup transactions that would otherwise inflate contributions, or other account totals, reported for the group as a single entity (in effect, preventing double reporting of contributions or other items).

COMBINED FINANCIAL STATEMENTS: A CASE STUDY

This section is presented to provide additional guidance in helping organizations decide whether or not it is appropriate to issue combined financial statements for the reporting entity and its affiliates. The following compares factors that indicate control vs. factors that suggest lack of control, in an outline form.

Factors Related to Control

Factors related to control which may indicate that the Affiliated Organization ("A") should be combined with the Reporting Organization ("R"), if other criteria for combination are met. Note that many of these factors are not determinative by themselves, but should be considered in conjunction with other factors.

CONTROL

Organization relationship

— A is clearly described as controlled by, for the benefit of, or an affiliate of R in some of the following:

- articles/charter/by-laws
- operating/affiliation agreement
- fund-raising material/membership brochure
- annual report
- grant proposals
- application for tax-exempt status

LACK OF CONTROL

— A is described as independent of R, or no formal relationship is indicated

CONTROL	*LACK OF CONTROL*
Governance	
— A's board has a majority of its membership in common with R; common officers	— Little or no overlap
— A's board members and/or officers are appointed by R, or are subject to approval of R's board, officers, or members	— A's board is self-perpetuating (determining) with no input from R
— Major decisions of A's board, officers or staff are subject to review, approval, or ratification by R	— A's decisions are made autonomously; or even if in theory subject to such control, R has, in fact, never or rarely exercised control and does not intend to do so
Financial	
— A's budget is subject to review or approval by R	— Budget not subject to R's approval
— Some or all of A's disbursements are subject to approval or countersignature by R	— Checks may be issued without R's approval
— A's excess of revenue over expenses or fund balances, or portions thereof, are subject to being transferred to R at R's request, or are automatically transferred (by custom, contract or otherwise)	— Although some of A's financial resources may be transferred to R, this is done only at the discretion of A's board
— A's activities are largely financed by grants, loans or transfers from R, or from other sources determined by R's board	— A's activities are financed from sources determined by A's board
— A's by-laws indicate that its resources are intended to be used for activities similar to those of R	— A's by-laws limit uses of resources to purposes which do not include R's activities

CONTROL	*LACK OF CONTROL*
— A's fund-raising appeals give donors the impression that gifts will be used to further R's programs	— Appeals give the impression that funds will be used by A
— A and R submit combined financial data to funding sources, regulatory bodies, and other outside parties	— Separate data are submitted
Operating	
— A shares with R many of the following operating functions: • personnel/payroll • purchasing • professional services • fund raising • accounting, treasury • office space	— Few operating functions are shared; or reimbursement of costs is on a strictly arms-length basis with formal contracts
— Decisions about A's program or other activities are made by R or are subject to R's review or approval	— A's decisions are made autonomously
— A's activities are almost exclusively for the benefit of R's members or beneficiaries	— Activities benefit persons unaffiliated with R

CHAPTER VIII

ILLUSTRATIVE FINANCIAL STATEMENTS

The *Standards* provides uniform accounting and financial reporting procedures sufficiently detailed and extensive to meet the reporting needs, at one extreme, of small local agencies and, at the other, of very large national organizations. The preceding chapters have necessarily attempted to treat the wide variations in sources of support and revenue and types of net assets and balance sheet accounts of the different voluntary health and welfare organizations. Illustrative forms of financial statements for public reporting reflecting these accounting standards are presented in the following pages. They represent a single set of financial statements of a medium-sized, affiliated voluntary organization. In the preparation of combined financial statements for all affiliated entities of an organization, whether at the state or national level, transactions between the entities would be eliminated. Accordingly, the captions in Exhibits B and C regarding sharing of contributions, sales of materials and services, etc. would not appear in combined financial statements.

The revenue section of Exhibit B illustrates more accounts than an agency is likely to need. All organizations—of whatever size, whether at the local, state or national level, and whether affiliated or fully independent—may present statements simplified to meet their own requirements by the omission of those items not applicable to their operations. On the other hand, the accounts in earned revenue, expenses and other classifications may prove inadequate for some large and complex organizations. As previously suggested, organizations in designing their financial statements may choose to supplement or expand categories shown in the illustrated statements to suit their needs. At the same time, they should conform this supplementation and expansion with the classifications and categories of the illustrated statements.

Regardless of its size or the simplicity of its financial structure, every agency seeking to conform its annual financial reports to the *Standards* should include, in one report, at least the following three forms of statements and accompanying notes:

Balance Sheet,
Statement of Revenue and Expenses and Changes in Fund Balances, and
Statement of Functional Expenses.

The illustrated forms of Exhibits A and B are columnar. As to Exhibit A—the Balance Sheet, while a columnar presentation is illustrated, a layered format is also acceptable.

Expenses appearing on Exhibit B, in particular program services and supporting services, are derived from Exhibit C. In this regard, an explanation on the transposition of these expenses, including depreciation, from Exhibit C to Exhibit B, is provided in Chapter V.

The AICPA Voluntary Health and Welfare audit guide notes that a Statement of Changes in Financial Position is not generally required, since the information normally presented in such a statement is readily available in the Statement of Revenue and Expenses and Changes in Fund Balances. However, those agencies that wish to present such a statement or a Statement of Cash Flow may do so.

Agencies should include notes to their financial statements that provide any additional information needed for fair presentation, such as significant accounting policies, mortgage agreements, pension plans, contingent liabilities, etc. In every case, the standard of public financial reporting to follow is to report all significant facts necessary to make an organization's financial statements fully informative and not misleading. It is thus considered desirable (and in many states required) that, to fulfill its obligation to the contributing public, the accounts of a voluntary health or welfare organization be examined annually, in accordance with generally accepted accounting principles by independent auditors.

Voluntary agencies should include in their published financial statements separate columns showing comparative data for the preceding year. Their repetition in an agency's current statements may be expected to improve a reader's understanding of the report and his or her grasp of its significance. When using a columnar format, presentation of only the prior year total column will often be sufficient for this purpose.

It should be noted that the amounts shown in the accompanying statements have been included for illustrative purposes only. No attempt has been made to conform them to relationships exhibited by financial data of any group of voluntary agencies or to suggest particular relationships. Modifications to the illustrated financial statements should be made to fit the facts and circumstances of each specific organization.

It should also be noted that while previous editions of *Standards* presented the Statement of Revenue and Expenses and Changes in Fund Balance as the first statement, the recommended presentation has been changed to present the Balance Sheet first, to conform with the general practice of other not-for-profit organizations.

NOTE: For illustrated financial statements of United Ways and Federated Fund-Raising Organizations, see Appendix 2, pp. 108–113.

EXHIBIT A

VOLUNTARY HEALTH AND WELFARE SERVICE AFFILIATE

Balance Sheet

	For the Year Ended December 31,					
	19X2					19X1
	Current Funds		Land, Building and Equipment Fund	Endowment Fund	Total	Total
ASSETS	Unrestricted	Restricted				
Current assets:						
Cash, including $115,000 and $123,000 in interest-bearing accounts	$121,100	$ 300			$121,400	$127,000
Short-term investments, at cost (approximates market)	100,000	7,100			107,100	121,700
Receivables:						
Program service fees, less allowance of $200 and $100	600				600	800
Pledges, less allowance of $11,200 and $9,700	58,900				58,900	46,000
Grants		1,000	$ 4,800		5,800	4,600
From affiliated organizations	1,000				1,000	1,000
Interfund receivable (payable)	2,000	(2,000)				
Inventory, at lower of cost or market	7,000				7,000	6,100
Prepaid expenses and deferred charges	13,800				13,800	9,600
Total current assets	304,400	6,400	4,800		315,600	316,800
Non-current investments (Note 3)	279,600			$194,800	474,400	430,700
Land, buildings, and equipment, at cost, less accumulated depreciation (Note 6)			174,800		174,800	168,500
Total assets	$584,000	$6,400	$179,600	$194,800	$964,800	$916,000

LIABILITIES AND FUND BALANCES						
Current liabilities:						
Accounts payable and accrued expenses	$ 39,300				$ 39,300	$ 46,000
Research grants (Note 4)	41,600				41,600	45,600
Support & revenue designated for subsequent period	18,000				18,000	16,000
Total current liabilities	98,900				98,900	107,600
Mortgage payable, 6%, due 19XX (Note 12)			$ 3,200		3,200	3,600
Amounts payable under capital lease (Note 10)			10,200		10,200	
Total liabilities	98,900		13,400		112,300	111,200
Fund balances:						
Current unrestricted:						
Designated by the governing board for—						
Long-term investment	279,600				279,600	239,000
Purchase of new equipment	10,400				10,400	
Research purposes (Note 4)	115,200				115,200	175,800
Undesignated—available for general activities	79,900				79,900	31,500
Current restricted for:						
Professional education		$4,000			4,000	
Research grants		2,400			2,400	10,000
Land, building and equipment fund:						
Unexpended restricted (Note 5)			4,800		4,800	2,100
Equity in fixed assets			161,400		161,400	154,700
Endowment fund				$194,800	194,800	191,700
Total fund balances	485,100	6,400	166,200	194,800	852,500	804,800
Total liabilities and fund balances	$584,000	$6,400	$179,600	$194,800	$964,800	$916,000

EXHIBIT B

VOLUNTARY HEALTH AND WELFARE SERVICE AFFILIATE

Statement of Revenue and Expenses and Changes in Fund Balances

	For the Year Ended December 31,					
	19X2					19X1
	Current Funds		Land, Building and Equipment Fund	Endowment Fund	Total	Total
	Unrestricted	Restricted				
Revenue:						
Public support—						
Received directly—						
Contributions (net of estimated uncollectible pledges of $19,500 and $15,000)........	$660,100	$ 6,200	$ 7,200	$ 200	$673,700	$700,400
Special events (net of costs of direct benefit to participants of $18,000 and $16,300)	10,400				10,400	9,200
Legacies and bequests....................	9,200			400	9,600	12,000
Donated services (Note 7)	8,000				8,000	7,000
Received indirectly—						
Collected through local member units.......	4,000				4,000	7,900
Allocated by federated fund-raising organizations (net of their related fund-raising expenses estimated at $2,300 and $2,200)	23,500				23,500	22,000
Total public support	715,200	6,200	7,200	600	729,200	758,500
Revenue and grants from governmental agencies		300			300	300
Other revenue:						
Membership dues—individuals	500				500	400
Assessments and dues—local member units ...	1,100				1,100	700

Program service fees	2,300				2,300	800
Sales of materials and services (net of direct expenses of $1,000 and $700)	400				400	300
Endowment and other investment income	30,500	700			31,200	26,000
Miscellaneous revenue	2,800				2,800	3,600
Gains (losses) on investments	(2,000)			2,500	500	27,500
Total other revenue	35,600	700		2,500	38,800	59,300
Total revenue	750,800	7,200	7,200	3,100	768,300	818,100
Expenses:						
Program services—						
Program A	141,200		200		141,400	136,500
Program B	53,900		500		54,400	48,500
Program C	61,200		600		61,800	51,600
Program D	244,100	10,800	2,900		257,800	273,600
Total program services	500,400	10,800	4,200		515,400	510,200
Supporting services—						
Management and general	56,800		600		57,400	63,800
Fund-raising	65,000		400		65,400	54,600
Total supporting services	121,800		1,000		122,800	118,400
Payments to national organization (Note 11)	82,400				82,400	85,400
Total expenses	704,600	10,800	5,200		720,600	714,000
Excess (deficiency) of revenue over expenses	46,200	(3,600)	2,000	3,100	47,700	104,100
Fund balances, beginning of year	446,300	10,000	156,800	191,700	804,800	700,700
Other changes in fund balances:						
Acquisition of fixed assets	(7,000)		7,000			
Mortgage Payment	(400)		400			
Fund Balances, end of year	$485,100	$ 6,400	$166,200	$194,800	$852,500	$804,800

EXHIBIT C

VOLUNTARY HEALTH AND WELFARE SERVICE AFFILIATE

Statement of Functional Expenses

For the Year ended December 31, 19X2 with Comparative Totals for 19X1

	Program Services					Supporting Services			Total Program and Supporting Services Expenses	
	Program A	Program B	Program C	Program D	Total	Management and General	Fund Raising	Total	19X2	19X1
Salaries	$ 4,500	$29,100	$25,100	$126,900	$185,600	$33,100	$36,800	$ 69,900	$255,500	$243,300
Employee benefits	400	1,400	1,400	6,400	9,600	2,200	1,500	3,700	13,300	12,500
Payroll taxes, etc.	400	2,600	2,300	12,400	17,700	3,000	3,100	6,100	23,800	21,500
Total salaries and related expenses	5,300	33,100	28,800	145,700	212,900	38,300	41,400	79,700	292,600	277,300

Professional fees	—	1,000	300	1,200	2,500	2,600	800	3,400	5,900	5,300
Supplies	600	1,300	1,300	1,300	4,500	1,800	1,700	3,500	8,000	7,100
Telephone	200	300	1,000	1,100	2,600	1,500	2,300	3,800	6,400	6,800
Postage and shipping	200	1,700	1,300	8,900	12,100	1,000	9,000	10,000	22,100	8,000
Occupancy	250	1,300	1,100	1,250	3,900	1,500	1,350	2,850	6,750	6,300
Interest	—	—	—	100	100	800	—	800	900	200
Rental and maintenance of equipment	250	1,300	1,100	1,250	3,900	1,500	1,350	2,850	6,750	6,300
Printing and publications	—	2,400	400	6,400	9,200	300	1,600	1,900	11,100	5,800
Travel and transportation	300	2,200	2,000	2,200	6,700	2,300	3,000	5,300	12,000	11,300
Conferences, conventions & meetings	800	1,900	7,100	2,000	11,800	4,500	400	4,900	16,700	15,600
Specific assistance to individuals	—	6,500	4,300	—	10,800	—	—	—	10,800	18,400
Membership dues	—	500	—	—	500	—	—	—	500	500
Awards and grants—										
To National Organization	—	—	—	83,000	83,000	—	—	—	83,000	104,200
To individuals and other organizations	133,200	—	11,900	—	145,100	—	—	—	145,100	144,300
Insurance	50	200	100	100	450	600	50	650	1,100	1,000
Other expenses	50	200	500	400	1,150	100	2,050	2,150	3,300	5,600
Depreciation of buildings & equipment	200	500	600	2,900	4,200	600	400	1,000	5,200	4,600
Total functional expenses:	$141,400	$54,400	$61,800	$257,800	$515,400	$57,400	$65,400	$122,800	638,200	628,600
Payments to National Organization									82,400	85,400
Total expenses									$720,600	$714,000

VOLUNTARY HEALTH AND WELFARE SERVICE AFFILIATE

NOTES TO FINANCIAL STATEMENTS DECEMBER 31, 19X2

1. *Description of Organization*—The Voluntary Health and Welfare Service Affiliate, a nonprofit organization, is a local unit of the National Voluntary Health and Welfare Service. Its principal programs include: Research—financial support provided to academic institutions and scientists seeking knowledge of the causes, cures and prevention of ________ disease; Public Health Education—programs designed to promote effective health practices; Professional Health Education—programs designed to improve the knowledge and skills of the medical and allied professions in the prevention, detection and diagnosis and treatment of patients; and Community Health Services—services provided for conduct of rehabilitation and other patient programs, planning and improving community health practices, supporting clinics and other health facilities. The Service also cooperates and assists in the local fund-raising activities of the national organization.

   The Service is exempt from income tax under Section 501(c)(3) of the U.S. Internal Revenue Code and comparable State law, and contributions to it are tax deductible within the limitations prescribed by the Code. The Service has been classified as a publicly-supported organization which is not a private foundation under Section 509(a) of the Code.

2. *Significant Accounting Policies*—All contributions are considered available for unrestricted use, unless specifically restricted by the donor. Pledges are recorded in the Balance Sheet when the agency is notified of the pledge, and allowances are provided for amounts estimated as uncollectible. Bequests are recorded as income at the time the Service has an established right to the bequest and the proceeds are measurable. Additional accounting policies are included in other footnotes. [Some organizations may wish to present all accounting policies in this footnote.]

3. *Investments*—Investments in marketable common stocks and bonds are reported at cost. Market values and unrealized appreciation (depreciation) at December 31, 19X2 are summarized as follows:

	December 31, 19X2	
	Quoted Market Value	Unrealized Appreciation
Unrestricted Board-designated long-term investments:		
Common stocks	$160,000	$10,000
Corporate bonds	134,600	5,000
	$294,600	$15,000
Endowment:		
Investment cash	$ 400	—

Common stocks	113,000	$ 3,000
Corporate bonds	86,400	2,000
	$199,800	$ 5,000

4. *Awards and Grants*—The Service's awards and grants are recorded when voted by its governing board.

5. *Proposed Research Center*—The XYZ Foundation has contributed $4,800 to the Service with the stipulations that it be used for the construction of a research center and that the construction of the facilities begin within four years. The Service is considering the construction of a research center, the cost of which would approximate $200,000. If the governing board approves the construction of these facilities, it is contemplated that its cost would be financed by a special fund drive.

6. *Land, Buildings, Equipment and Depreciation*—The Service follows the practice of capitalizing all expenditures for land, buildings and equipment in excess of $500; the fair value of donated fixed assets is similarly capitalized. Depreciation of buildings and equipment is provided on a straight-line basis over the estimated useful lives of the assets (2 percent per year for buildings, 10 percent for medical research equipment and office furniture and equipment, and 33 percent for the automobile). At December 31, 19X2 such assets were:

	19X2
Land	$ 37,600
Buildings	100,000
Medical research equipment	33,600
Office furniture and equipment	24,600
Automobile	8,000
Total	203,800
Less accumulated depreciation	29,000
	$174,800

7. *Donated Materials and Services*—Donated materials and equipment are reflected as contributions in the accompanying statements at their estimated values at date of receipt. The value of donated services is recorded as contributions and salary expense in the period rendered.
OR
[No amounts have been reflected in the statements for donated services, since no objective basis is available to measure the value of such services. Nevertheless, a substantial number of volunteers have donated significant amounts of their time in the organization's program services and its fund-raising campaigns.]

8. *Pension Plan*—The Service has a defined benefit pension plan covering substantially all of its employees. The benefits are based on years of service and the employee's compensation during the last five years of employment. The funding policy is to fund pension cost accrued. Contributions are intended to

provide not only for benefits attributed to service to date, but also for those expected to be earned in the future.

The following table sets forth the plan's funded status and amounts recognized in the balance sheet at December 31, 19X2:

Actuarial present value of benefit obligations:	
Accumulated benefit obligation, including vested benefits of $2,870	$(3,350)
Projected benefit obligation for service rendered to date	$(5,000)
Plan assets at fair value, primarily listed stocks and U.S. bonds	4,750
Projected benefit obligation in excess of plan assets	(250)
Unrecognized net gain from past experience different from that assumed and effects of changes in assumptions	(530)
Prior service cost not yet recognized in net periodic pension cost	190
Unrecognized net obligation at January 1, 1986 being recognized over 15 years	770
Prepaid pension cost included in deferred charges	$ 180

Net pension cost included the following components:

	19X2
Service cost (benefits earned during the period)	$260
Interest cost on projected benefit obligation	390
Actual return on plan assets	(450)
Net amortization and deferral	100
Net periodic pension cost	$300

The weighted-average discount rate and rate of increase in future compensation levels used in determining the actuarial present value of the projected benefit obligation were 7 percent and 5 percent, respectively, in both years. The expected long-term rate of return on assets was 8 percent in 19X2.

The Service has a defined contribution retirement plan covering substantially all of its employees. The Service matches each employee's contribution to the plan, with each employee's contribution being limited to a percentage of salary. Contributions by the Service are fully vested to the employees on the contribution date. The retirement plan contribution included in expenses was $300 in 19X2.

9. *Other Post-Retirement Benefits*—The Service provides certain health care and life insurance benefits for retired employees. Substantially all of the employees may become eligible for this benefit if they reach normal retirement age while still working for the Service. Those benefits and similar benefits for active employees are provided through insurance companies whose premiums are based on the benefits paid during the year. The Service recognized the cost of

providing those benefits by expensing the annual insurance premiums, which were $3,044 in 19X2. Of this amount, $960 was applicable to retirees.

10. *Lease Commitments*—The Service rents certain office equipment under a capital lease, expiring in 19X9. Payments under this lease are as follows:

19X3–19X8 at $2,000 per year	$12,000
19X9	700
Total lease payments	12,700
Less amount representing interest	2,500
Present value of lease payments	$10,200

The following is a schedule, by years, of the approximate future minimum rental payments required under operating leases that have initial or remaining noncancelable lease terms in excess of one year as of December 31, 19X2:

Fiscal Years	
19X3	$ 3,000
19X4	3,000
19X5	3,000
19X6	2,000
19X7	3,000
later, to 2002	30,000

Rental expense aggregated approximately $5,000 in 19X2.

11. *Sharing of Public Support*—In accordance with the affiliation agreement with the national organization, 12 percent of most unrestricted support from the public is remitted to the national organization for its use as determined by its board of directors. Additional grants are made as determined by the Service Affiliate's board of directors; these amounts being shown as awards and grants in the Statement of Functional Expenses.

12. *Mortgage*—The mortgage is secured by the Service's land and buildings. It is payable in monthly installments to the State Bank.

13. *Allocation to Joint Information Costs*—In 19X2, the Service incurred joint costs of $9,600 for informational materials and activities that included fund-raising appeals. Of those costs, $6,100 was allocated to fund-raising expense, $400 was allocated to Program B expense, $2,400 was allocated to Program D expense, and $700 was allocated to management and general expense.

appendix I

METHODS OF EXPENSE ALLOCATION

The functional expense accounting standards described in Chapter V require voluntary health and welfare organizations to maintain records that reflect the classification of expenses both as to object and function. This Appendix examines the kind of expense accounting called for in Chapter V to promote uniformity in application and to minimize additional work in complying with the *Standards*.

FUNCTIONAL ACCOUNTING PRACTICES FOR PUBLIC REPORTING

Voluntary health and welfare organizations vary greatly in size, complexity of their activities and staff resources. Thousands of small agencies are administered entirely by volunteers. Each agency must adapt its accounting operation to its own activities, organization and staff resources. The following paragraphs suggest a practical approach to functional accounting adequate for public financial reporting.

In developing its functional accounting procedures, agencies should consult with their independent auditors, who must determine the reasonableness of the distributions of functional expenses in order to render an unqualified opinion on the financial statements.

The methods described in this appendix will also be useful for other types of financial reporting—e.g., to government agencies, foundations, etc. For example, if a project supported by a government agency or a foundation is conducted within a functional classification that also includes other types of activities, the methods used to accumulate expenses at the "functional level" should also be used to accumulate costs at the "project level" in order to separate the project costs from those of other activities.

Recording Expenses by Function Whenever Possible

Whether expenses are recorded initially on a checkbook stub or in a multicolumn cash disbursements journal, the object expense account of each payment should be indicated at the time it is initially recorded—e.g., supplies, telephone—according to an agency's object expense classifications. To facilitate functional accounting for the same expenses, the functional expense account should be entered simultaneously with the object classification whenever possible. It will normally be possible to do so with respect to any expenses incurred for and benefiting only a single function—e.g., supplies for a camp, doctor's fee paid for a client in connection with a single health program. The evident benefits of such point-of-original-entry functional classification of direct expenses are: reduction of month-end analyses, minimization of possible incorrect classifications and establishment of direct documentary evidence supporting an agency's functional classifications.

Expenses Distributable to More Than One Function

The most difficult problem of accounting for expenses by function is posed by expenses that benefit more than one function—e.g., salaries, office rent, travel expenses. Organizations are required to develop techniques that will provide verifiable bases upon which expenses may be related to program or supporting service functions. Many expenses may logically be related to time spent on particular functions—e.g., salaries, travel expenses. Others vary with space used for particular functions: office rent, building depreciation, electricity, heat and janitorial supplies are obvious examples. The identification of equipment used in different functions may provide a logical basis for distributing related depreciation, maintenance, repairs and insurance expenses. If space-related expenses are to be distributed among services using a particular building, it will be necessary to determine the proportion of space used for each function—normally by measurement of floor areas occupied.

Distribution of expenses based on employees' time requires time analysis or time reporting, as will be discussed. Other bases for distribution of expenses may usually be established through a survey, as of space used for different functions, the results of which will furnish a standard basis for distributing related expenses among functions. Agencies experiencing relatively frequent changes in their activities, staff, and facilities need to remain alert for changes sufficiently important to require reexamination of established expense-distribution bases. At a minimum, these studies should be updated annually.

TIME REPORTING FOR FUNCTIONAL EXPENSE ACCOUNTING

Since personal services constitute the largest single cost of most voluntary health and welfare organizations, accounting for staff members' time spent in particular program and supporting services is essential for functional expense reporting by voluntary agencies. For employees whose time is spent exclusively on activities of one program or supporting service, no time reporting problem exists; their compensation and related expenses such as payroll taxes and employee benefit expenses may be charged directly to the particular service.

Functional expense distribution of compensation of staff members engaged in more than one service during an accounting period requires the accumulation of reliable data upon which such allocations can be made. In some instances, the activities of employees vary considerably throughout the year and from year to year, and thus only the daily time sheet will reasonably reflect the functional distribution. However, accumulation of daily detail time reports for all employees is not required in all instances. Rather, periodic testing of the actual work done by employees in representative job classifications may provide the data needed to determine allocations. The determination and use of a sample distribution does, however, require great care. The periods selected for sampling must be both sufficiently random and of sufficient duration to be statistically representative of an employee's total activities for the year reported upon. In most cases, this will require that sampling procedures be established on a continuing basis. Whether time reports are kept on a full-time basis or tests made of sample periods, guidelines should be established reflecting anticipated activities against which the results of the actual time reports may be measured for reasonableness. Employees must be trained in the procedures to be followed in time reporting, and the appropriate functional classification of each of their normal tasks should be discussed with them in advance. In addition, provision should be made for continual monitoring of the time reporting program to detect and correct errors.

INVOLVEMENT OF MANAGEMENT

The functional classification of expenses permits an agency to tell the reader of the financial statements not only the nature of its expenses, but also the purpose for which they were made. Accordingly, it can never be considered solely a bookkeeping matter. Rather, the agency's management must ensure that the techniques used in accumulating such cost data are adequate and that the results, as reflected in the financial statements, fairly present the actual operations for the year.

A RECOMMENDED PROCEDURE FOR FUNCTIONAL ALLOCATION OF SALARY EXPENSES

The following paragraphs illustrate a procedure that has proved workable and is recommended, where applicable, for adoption by voluntary agencies.

At the time the annual budget is prepared, employees expected to spend their entire time working in one function during the coming year should be identified. Since salaries of these people should be charged directly to the applicable functions, no time sheets are required. However, to assure that their assignments have not changed, a regular, periodic review should be made of their duties and a note entered in the functional allocation documentation that this has been done.

Also at budget time, employees expected to perform work in several functions should be identified. The duties of each employee should then be reviewed and a summary job description prepared, listing both the nature and functional classification of work to be done, and the approximate time to be spent in the respective areas during the coming year. This document should reflect the job tasks in sufficient detail to serve as a reference source for determining proper functional allocations by the employee when preparing time reports. Budgeted allocation percentages should next be prepared for each employee on the basis of this review, together with an understanding of the actual nature of the work to be done as determined by knowledgeable supervisory personnel. In the event that the functional allocation of compensation is to be reflected in the interim financial statements, such allocations may be made on the basis of these budgeted percentages. The reliability of the budgeted allocation percentages should be verified by a continuing test program of time reporting described below.

Time Reports

Selected employees should be required to submit time reports. In the case of larger organizations, it may be satisfactory to identify representative individuals in each job category, rather than requiring all employees to submit reports.

Frequency of Reports

Time reports of these selected individuals should be required on a regular basis. In most cases, reporting of activities during one week of each month will provide the necessary information to determine whether the work being done is in accordance with that anticipated in the budget and will, at the same time, adequately reflect the results of seasonal patterns in work assignments. To assure that the periods are representative, a different week of the month should be selected on a rotating basis.

Staff Training

The individuals designated to submit time reports should be instructed in their preparation. This involves not only a clear understanding of the mechanics of the forms but, more importantly, an adequate understanding of which functions, in an accounting and financial reporting sense, benefit from their individual activities. It is particularly important in this effort that employees recognize that administration of programs and fund-raising activities should be charged to those functions and not to management and general.

Report Contents

The time reports should include a brief description of the actual tasks performed, as well as the functions which benefited, and the number of hours spent on each function. Normally, allocation of time to the nearest hour will provide sufficient accuracy for this purpose. All time worked should be accounted for, including overtime and travel time.

Signing and Supervision

Each time report should be reviewed promptly and signed by a supervisor to assure that an examination of the reports has been made for accuracy and representativeness.

Work Sheets Summary

These reports should be summarized on work sheets by an employee. At year-end, the work sheets should be summarized to reflect the total hours and percentages of aggregate time for which reports were submitted, by function, for comparison with the predetermined estimated percentages established at the time the budget was prepared.

Comparison of Actual Percentages

In the event significant variations exist between overall actual percentages and those determined at the time of budget preparation, an investigation should be made and documented to determine the reasons for the variations. If, for example, the assigned duties differ from those that were planned, then it should be determined whether the actual results were representative of the work assigned to all employees in the particular job category. If this is the case, then the predetermined estimates should be revised as appropriate to reflect the actual work done. These revised rates should be used in making the final allocations for the financial statements.

Samples

Sample time reports and related work sheets are shown at the end of this appendix.

Summary

Obviously, the allocation of salary costs requires the exercise of judgment. The involvement of key management personnel is essential to avoid a strictly mechanical approach which would result in allocations that do not fairly reflect the actual activities of the organization. It is also essential that there be adequate planning, careful selection and training of employees who submit time reports, and checks on the actual results to ensure that they are reasonable in light of the agency's actual activities.

Daily Time Record

Name: ______________________________

Job Title: ______________________________

Date: ______________________________

Description of Work Done	Function Benefited*	Number of Hours
____________________	Research	______
____________________		
____________________	Public Education	______
____________________		
____________________	Professional Education & Training	______
____________________		
____________________	Patient Services	______
____________________		
____________________	Community Services	______
____________________		
____________________	Management & General	______
____________________		
____________________	Fund Raising	______
____________________		
	TOTAL HOURS WORKED	______

____

Supervisor Approval

*These are the program services categories generally utilized by various health agencies and are cited here for illustrative purposes. Thousands of relatively small, single program/purpose organizations will need to functionalize expenses in only three categories: (1) Program Service; (2) Management and General; and (3) Fund Raising.

Annual Time Allocation Summary

Name: ______________________________

Job Title: ______________________________

Week Beginning	Total Hours	Research	Public Education	Professional Education & Training	Patient Services	Community Services	Management & General	Fund Raising
Annual Hours								
Actual %								
Estimated %								
Difference								

appendix 2

SPECIAL STANDARDS FOR FUND-RAISING AND FUND-DISTRIBUTION ACTIVITIES OF UNITED WAYS (UW) AND FEDERATED FUND-RAISING ORGANIZATIONS (FFO)

Certain problems of financial reporting are unique to United Ways (also known as United Fund, Community Chest, United Appeal, etc.) and federated fund-raising organizations [FFO]. While these organizations should observe the same financial reporting standards as other voluntary organizations, they may encounter difficulties in reporting—in a single set of financial statements—the support, revenue and expenses incurred over several years, and in classifying expenses by program and supporting services.

By FFO is meant community and other voluntary organizations that perform all of the following primary activities:

1. Campaign for contributions, for the benefit of two or more voluntary health and/or welfare organizations, within designated geographical, religious, industrial or other communities.
2. Review requests of affiliates or other organizations seeking funding or participation in a federated fund-raising drive, as provided for in the agreement between the FFO and its participants.
3. Distribute funds to these organizations on the basis of approved budgets or requests, community needs, or other participation agreements and arrangements.

The following additional terms are used in this appendix with the special meanings shown:

Term	*Special Meaning*
Distribution	The amount formally approved or otherwise determined by a UW or FFO as funding for a particular organization during the distribution year (defined below).

Annual Campaign	A community-wide or other campaign for funds, initiated by a United Way or FFO once a year and identified with the distribution year—e.g., "the 1986 Annual Campaign" would refer to the campaign conducted in 1985 for funds to be distributed for 1986.
Campaign Period	The period of time between the start of the planning, promotion, and initiation of appeals for contributions and pledges, under a particular annual campaign, and its formal termination date, where applicable.
Campaign Production	The total dollar value of contributions and pledges received and receivable by a UW or FFO as the result of a given annual campaign.
Distribution year	The 12-month period for which a UW or FFO earmarks all (or substantially all) of its distributions from a given year's campaign.
Promotion Period	The period over which all of the expenses of promotion of a particular annual campaign are incurred.

What makes United Ways and FFOs different for financial reporting purposes is that, to the extent practical, they need to emphasize in their reports for each year the financial transactions—namely, total amount raised, total amount distributed and the expenses related to the amount raised—which generally take place over two or more years. The promotion period may begin as much as a year before a given annual campaign. Post-campaign revised-budget reviews and distribution may last several months beyond the campaign period.

The accounting procedures suggested under these circumstances for United Ways and FFOs in their annual financial reports to the public are based on the concept of "matching" and are summarized below:

1. These organizations should, insofar as is practical, have their fiscal year coincide with their distribution year.
2. Fund-raising expenses for a given annual campaign should be reported as prepaid expenses until the distribution year, at which point they should be reported as campaign expenses.
3. The amount raised from the given annual campaign should be reported as deferred support until the following distribution year. Then it should be reported as support.
4. Distributions made from the annual campaign production before the distribution year should be charged against deferred campaign support and reported parenthetically as follows—or as prepaid distributions, as in Exhibit X: Annual campaign support designated for future periods (net of advance distributions to agencies of $X).

   For the distribution year, campaign support should be reported as gross distributions whether or not they had been previously deferred.

The techniques outlined defer the reporting of the entire fund-raising expenses, production and distribution of a given annual campaign to be reported in the Statement of Revenue and Expenses and Changes in Fund Balances of the distribution year. This treatment will not only match in a single statement the reporting of activities properly related, but should also simplify internal budgeting and distribution control. It will permit uniform financial reporting both by an organization with a long promotion period, and by an organization whose distributions and campaign production are incomplete until after the start of its distribution year. It will show the contributor, in a single statement for any such organization, the production, distribution and fund-raising expenses of each annual campaign.

It is recognized that the procedures described above, while conceptually sound, may not be practical for all United Ways and FFOs. In fact, since the publication of *Standards* in 1964, and its revision in 1974, some of these organizations are reported to have found it inappropriate to utilize these techniques because of the absence of distinct relationships between the fund-raising and fund-distribution periods and the timing of these activities. With these exceptions noted, however, all UWs and FFOs should adopt the above procedures, as appropriate.

CLASSIFYING ACTIVITIES AS PROGRAM OR SUPPORT

Since most of the activities for which funds are raised by these organizations are conducted by others—i.e., the agencies to which funds are given—the classification of expenses as program services or supporting services takes on a special meaning.

In the case of United Ways, "fund raising" is one of the primary services provided to donors, agencies and the community at large, and, for that reason, is considered by them and those benefiting, a major "program service." With respect to the FFOs, the same logic prevails. The name—federated fundraising organization—itself says it. In fact, most if not all FFOs perform the primary service of raising funds for a group of like organizations and then, as a rule, distribute the dollars according to some predetermined formula or agreement. Thus, for United Ways and FFOs, it would be inaccurate to call their fund-raising service a "supporting service."

Regardless of the issue of classification (program vs. support), however, it is essential that these organizations reflect separately in their annual year-end financial statements the total amounts distributed to other organizations, and the expenses incurred in: (1) fund raising, (2) fund distribution and related activities, and (3) management and general. In addition, where distinct services are provided either directly or indirectly to the public or to other organizations, they should be listed separately along with the expenses incurred for those services. For example, many UWs will list the following as separate items where expenses are material: (1) Community Problem Solving, (2) Social/Community Needs Assessment, (3) Information and Referral or First Call For Help, (4) Volunteer Bureau or Voluntary Action Center, and (5) Management Consultation and Technical Assistance. Where expenses for individual programs listed above are not significant, they may be totaled under the general caption of "Community Services" as displayed on Exhibit Y.

A special set of illustrative financial statements (Exhibits X, Y, and Z) applicable to United Ways are presented at the end of this Appendix. It will be noted that in the functional classification, expenses are not to be grouped as program services and supporting services. Instead, expense categories should be listed, where appropriate, as illustrated below:

DISTRIBUTIONS and EXPENSES	
Allocations, Grants, Designations and Other Distributions......	$XXXXX
Payments to Affiliated Organizations........................	XXXXX
Functional Expenses:	
Management and General................................	XXXXX
Fund Raising..	XXXXX
Fund Distribution and Related Activities.....................	XXXX
Community Services—	
Community Problem Solving..............................	XXXX
Social/Community Needs Assessment.......................	XXXX
Information and Referral................................	XXXX
Volunteer Bureau..	XXXX
Management Consultation and Technical Assistance..........	XXXX

Exhibit Y displays a summary line item "Community Services" as one of the functional expense categories, while Exhibit Z displays a breakout of five specific program services and related expenses with a total for "Community Services." Further, some United Ways and FFOs may engage in substantial program-related "public education" activities. In such instances, if material, "public education" expenses should be separately displayed in Exhibit Y and/or Z and listed under "Community Services."

Finally, it is also permissible and appropriate, where material and feasible, to disclose, via an additional schedule or exhibit to the financial statements, a listing of the names of the organizations to which distributions have been made and the related amount of each such distribution.

EXHIBIT X

UNITED WAY OF UTOPIA, INC.

Balance Sheet

ASSETS	For the Year Ended December 31, 19X2: Current Funds Unrestricted	Current Funds Restricted	Land, Building and Equipment Fund	Endowment Fund	Total	19X1 Total
Cash, including $283,000 and $229,000 in interest-bearing accounts	$ 296,264	$ 62,858	$ 62,732		$ 421,854	$ 299,006
Short-term investments, at cost (approximates market)	5,100,000	100,000		$ 91,915	5,291,915	4,500,000
Receivables:						
Annual campaign, less allowance of $745,000 and $648,000	8,286,109				8,286,109	7,736,938
Capital loans to agencies	50,000				50,000	15,000
Grants		86,405			86,405	
Interfund receivable (payable)	6,000		(6,000)			
Prepaid expenses and deferred charges	43,229				43,229	38,707
Prepaid campaign expenses	894,035				894,035	754,324
Prepaid distributions	660,000				660,000	582,000
Investments (Note)	111,577			853,151	964,728	872,920
Land, building and equipment at cost, less accumulated depreciation (Note)			1,411,793		1,411,793	1,385,672
Total assets	$15,447,214	$249,263	$1,468,525	$945,066	$18,110,068	$16,184,567

LIABILITIES, DEFERRED REVENUE AND FUND BALANCES						
Accounts payable and accrued expenses	$ 236,807	$ 12,682			$ 249,489	$ 164,328
Distributions payable	77,313				77,313	21,960
Annual campaign support designated for subsequent campaign year, less allowance for uncollectible pledges of $745,000 and $648,000	11,672,137				11,672,137	10,158,512
Amounts payable under capital leases (Note)			$ 133,481		133,481	144,061
Mortgage payable (Note)			473,306		473,306	498,318
Annual campaign support designated for future periods	1,355,000				1,355,000	1,118,600
Total liabilities and deferred revenue	13,341,257	12,682	606,787		13,960,726	12,105,779
Fund balances:						
Current unrestricted:						
Designated by the governing board for—						
Long-term investment	111,577				111,577	111,577
Emergency reserve	1,800,000				1,800,000	1,800,000
Purchase of new equipment	100,000				100,000	100,000
Capital loans	50,000				50,000	50,000
Undesignated—available for general activities	44,380				44,380	80,792
Current restricted for:						
Venture grants		50,000			50,000	50,000
Information and referral		186,581			186,581	178,179
Land, building and equipment fund:						
Unexpended restricted			62,732		62,732	29,612
Equity in fixed assets			799,006		799,006	770,413
Endowment fund				$945,066	945,066	908,215
Total fund balances	2,105,957	236,581	861,738	945,066	4,149,342	4,078,788
Total liabilities, deferred revenue and fund balances	$15,447,214	$249,263	$1,468,525	$945,066	$18,110,068	$16,184,567

EXHIBIT Y

UNITED WAY OF UTOPIA, INC.

Statement of Revenue and Expenses and Changes in Fund Balances

	For the Year Ended December 31,					
	19X2					19X1
	Current Funds		Land, Building and Equipment Fund	Endowment Fund	Total	Total
	Unrestricted	Restricted				
Revenue:						
Public support received directly—						
Annual campaign (net of estimated uncollectible pledges of $648,000 and $564,700)	$10,158,512				$10,158,512	$8,846,960
Special events (net of costs of direct benefits to participants of $39,200 and $28,500)	45,758				45,758	36,111
Legacies and bequests	62,500				62,500	39,020
Donated services (Note)	17,000				17,000	8,000
Total public support	10,283,770				10,283,770	8,930,091
Revenue and grants from governmental agencies	—	$125,000			125,000	60,000
Other revenue:						
Program service fees	46,895				46,895	31,411
Investment income	165,209				165,209	142,237
Miscellaneous revenue	14,560				14,560	6,085
Gain (loss) on investment transactions	—	—		$ 36,,851	36,851	(12,297)
Total other revenue	226,664	—		36,851	263,515	167,436
Total revenue	10,510,434	125,000		36,851	10,672,285	9,157,527

Distributions and expenses:						
Allocations, grants, designations and other distributions	8,681,475				8,681,475	7,434,873
Payments to affiliated organizations	114,500				114,500	98,700
Functional expenses:						
Community services	392,537	116,598	$ 15,537		524,672	458,575
Management and general	410,136		9,601		419,737	362,852
Fund raising	740,952		15,533		756,485	657,816
Fund distribution	102,800		2,062		104,862	91,040
Total functional expenses	1,646,425	116,598	42,733		1,805,756	1,570,283
Total distributions and expenses	10,442,400	116,598	42,733		10,601,731	9,103,856
Excess (deficiency) of revenue over distributions and expenses	68,034	8,402	(42,733)	36,851	70,554	53,671
Fund balances, beginning of year	2,142,369	228,179	800,025	908,215	4,078,788	4,025,117
Other changes in fund balances:						
Acquisition of fixed assets	(68,854)		68,854			
Capital lease payments	(10,580)		10,580			
Mortgage payment	(25,012)		25,012			
Fund balances, end of year	$ 2,105,957	$236,581	$861,738	$945,066	$ 4,149,342	$4,078,788

EXHIBIT Z

UNITED WAY OF UTOPIA, INC.

Statement of Functional Expenses
Year Ended December 31, 19X2 With Comparative Totals For 19X1

	Community Services									Total	
	Community Problem Solving	Social/ Community Needs Assessment	Information and Referral	Volunteer Bureau	Management Consultation and Technical Assistance	Total	Management and General	Fund Raising	Fund Distribution	19X2	19X1
Salaries	$105,844	$17,400	$ 60,912	$28,300	$ 55,828	$268,284	$226,411	$391,960	$ 57,960	$ 944,615	$ 847,648
Employee benefits	28,518	3,448	10,043	7,399	14,879	64,287	51,621	85,647	13,732	215,287	188,666
Payroll taxes, etc.	6,737	1,253	5,465	1,318	3,660	18,433	16,302	28,941	4,336	68,012	61,030
Total salaries and related expenses	141,099	22,101	76,420	37,017	74,367	351,004	294,334	506,548	76,028	1,227,914	1,097,344
Professional fees	1,475	1,150				2,625	26,684	1,500		30,809	21,358
Supplies	5,809	3,883	1,210	1,154	2,330	14,386	6,872	13,467	1,250	35,975	26,077
Telephone	1,826	4,632	7,378	4,370	7,504	25,710	4,329	8,085	3,688	41,812	36,841
Postage and shipping	1,144	662	303	516	221	2,846	8,326	10,260	1,144	22,576	19,016
Occupancy	10,019	1,126	2,966	1,528	3,041	18,680	24,098	53,401	6,211	102,390	95,473
Interest	4,796	620	1,501	774	1,498	9,189	5,705	10,078	1,204	26,176	27,018
Rental and maintenance of equipment	2,809	5,618	1,238	1,079	2,616	13,360	4,722	6,537	2,687	27,306	20,553
Printing and publications	6,586	4,374	8,566	23,098	7,228	49,852	7,911	95,553	1,553	154,869	120,809
Travel and transportation	2,366	1,209	701	410	1,152	5,838	5,592	11,951	3,347	26,728	20,474
Conferences, conventions and meetings	2,156	4,033	976	711	1,255	9,131	7,674	8,419	3,988	29,212	22,315
Dues and subscriptions	558	277	421	565	417	2,238	3,661	2,472	715	9,086	8,856
Insurance	881	163	195	240	350	1,829	6,456	7,320	985	16,590	12,681
Other expenses		1,157		581	709	2,447	3,772	5,361		11,580	7,419
Depreciation of building and equipment	7,358	978	2,858	1,411	2,932	15,537	9,601	15,533	2,062	42,733	34,049

UNITED WAY OF UTOPIA, INC.

NOTES TO FINANCIAL STATEMENTS*
DECEMBER 31, 19X2

1. *Summary of Significant Accounting Policies*—Annual campaigns are conducted to raise support for allocation to participating agencies in the subsequent year. Campaigns conducted during the years ended December 31, 19X1 and 19X2 will be recognized in the years ended December 31, 19X2 and 19X3, respectively. Accordingly, campaign support and related expenses are deferred to the year of allocation to participating agencies. All support is considered available for unrestricted use unless specifically restricted by the donor. Pledges are recorded as received, and allowances are provided for amounts estimated as uncollectible.

*This note illustrates topics applicable to federated fund-raising organizations. Other information and notes are necessary and should generally parallel the notes to financial statements in Chapter VIII.

appendix 3

ILLUSTRATION OF AN INVESTMENT POOL

Three Funds (A, B and C) combined their cash some years ago into an investment pool by simultaneous contributions (in the portions indicated below) totaling $90,000, which was invested. On December 31, 19X5, the pooled investments on a cost basis were carried at $100,000, the original contributions plus $10,000 representing net realized gains retained by the investment pool.

The market value of the pooled assets was calculated to be $150,000. On this basis, the unrealized net gains are $50,000.

A new Fund (Fund D) puts $100,000 in cash into the investment pool at December 31, 19X5.

The following table presents the transactions set forth above and illustrates the calculation of the resulting equity percentages:

Fund	Cash Originally Contributed to Pool	Original Equity Percentage	Value of Pool on December 31, 19X5 Cost	Market	Value After Entry of Fund D	New Equity Percentage
A	$40,000	44.44%	$ 44,444	$ 66,667	$ 66,667	26.67%
B	35,000	38.89	38,889	58,333	58,333	23.33
C	15,000	16.67	16,667	25,000	25,000	10.00
D	—	—	—	—	100,000	40.00
	$90,000	100.00%	$100,000	$150,000	$250,000	100.00%

If Fund A were to withdraw from the investment pool at this date, it would be entitled to $66,667, rather than $44,444. The equity percentages to be used for entries to and withdrawals from the pool are based on market values, even though the accounting records may be kept on a cost basis.

appendix 4

EXAMPLE OF TRANSFER PROCEDURE RE: LAPSING OF TERM ENDOWMENT FUND RESTRICTION

An agency received a contribution of $100,000 that, by donor stipulation, is to be invested for a period of ten years, and only the income—i.e., interest and dividends—earned by the investments is to be used for general purposes of the agency. At the end of the ten-year period, the principal sum (as adjusted for appreciation and for depreciation, realized or unrealized) may be used by the agency for any of its related purposes.

In the year of receipt, the agency should report the contribution as public support in the Endowment Fund column of Exhibit B. The amount is also reflected as term endowment in the Endowment Fund of Exhibit A. Assuming that investments are carried at cost, gains and losses, as realized, would be reported in the other revenue section of Exhibit B in the Endowment Fund column. Interest and dividends from the investment would be included in the Current Unrestricted Fund as investment income.

If, at the end of the ten-year period stipulated by the donor, the invested contribution had a carrying value of $170,000 (as a result of net realized gains) and a market value of $200,000, it would be transferred from the Endowment Fund in the Other Changes in Fund Balances section of Exhibit B to the Current Unrestricted Fund in the amount of $200,000. A $30,000 gain would be reported in unrealized gains on investment transactions in Exhibit B in the Endowment Fund column.

appendix 5

INTERNAL CONTROL OVER CONTRIBUTIONS

All agencies have a responsibility to ensure that appropriate internal accounting controls are established and maintained over all categories of contributions. Simply defined, internal control is a system of procedures and cross-checking which, in the absence of collusion, both minimizes the likelihood of misappropriation of assets or misstatement of the accounts and maximizes the likelihood of prompt detection and assignment of responsibility if they do occur.

The objectives of internal accounting control for nonprofit organizations generally are the same as the objectives for profit-oriented organizations. Some characteristics of nonprofit organizations that influence internal accounting control include:

- A volunteer governing board, many of whose members serve for limited terms.
- A limited number of staff personnel, sometimes too few to provide the appropriate segregation of duties.
- A mixture of volunteers and employees participating in operations. Depending on the size and other features of the organization, day-to-day operations sometimes are conducted by volunteers instead of employees. The manner in which responsibility and authority are delegated varies among organizations. This may affect control over financial transactions, particularly with respect to authorization.
- A budget approved by the governing board. The budget may serve as authorization for the activities to be carried out by management in attaining the organization's program objectives. Nonprofit organizations should prepare budgets for both operating and capital expenditures.

Establishing internal control over contributions is often difficult, particularly where a gap exists between the time and place a contribution is originally made—e.g., to a door-to-door solicitor—and the time it is recorded in the books in the organization's office. Nevertheless, each agency must carefully consider its responsibility to establish appropriate internal controls. The AICPA Voluntary Health and Welfare audit guide requires the independent public accountant, who believes internal controls are not adequate, to issue a qualified opinion.

The audit guide discusses those internal control procedures normally appropriate over various types of contributions, including mail campaigns, door-to-door solicitation, street solicitation, etc. The audit guide notes, for instance, that "two employees should be assigned the function of jointly controlling incoming mail and preparing a record of amounts received . . . this record should be routinely compared with the bank deposits, preferably by someone not having access to the donations." Similar controls are indicated for other types of solicitation.

Each agency should discuss with its independent public accountant its system of internal accounting control over contributions to ensure that the agency is fulfilling its responsibilities. This will not only help to protect the agency but will also avoid placing the independent public accountant in the position of having to qualify the opinion due to inadequate internal controls. Also at stake is public confidence if it is disclosed that an agency does not employ reasonable and prudent safeguards in controlling contributed funds.

Summarized below are procedures that will assist agencies in establishing practical, cost-effective controls. The control procedures listed below are not intended to be all-inclusive or necessarily applicable to every situation. However, where basic sources of receipts exist, the procedures outlined can be adapted to just about any situation depending on the number of employees and type of existing control and accounting systems. Therefore, to the extent possible, the control procedures below should be implemented.

MAIL RECEIPTS

Effective control over mail receipts is essential. Control may be achieved by procedures such as the following:

— Joint control of mail received by the organization—Two or more persons (1) jointly control and open all incoming mail, (2) restrictively endorse checks immediately—including the number of the bank account in which the funds will be deposited, (3) prepare a list, in duplicate, of amounts received, (4) sign the list to attest to its accuracy, and (5) send one copy of the list to the organization's accounting department for recording in the accounting records, and send the second copy of the list, with the cash receipts, to the person responsible for making the bank deposit (who should be independent of the accounting function). A person who does not have access to cash receipts compares the bank deposit record with the accounting department cash receipts record.

— Use of a bank or other lock box service—The organization's fund-raising solicitations direct that contributions by mail be sent to a post office box. The recipient opens the mail, deposits the receipts, and furnishes the organization with a list of the lock box receipts and an authenticated deposit slip. If a lock box service is used, the organization should periodically ascertain that internal controls at the service are adequate and in effect. This may include requesting a letter to that effect from the independent auditor of the service. Also, prior to selection of a bank or "caging" operation to provide lock box services, an organization should ask for a current customer list so references can be checked, and should also request a tour of the operation to ensure that adequate controls exist.

The following procedures are sometimes used to supplement internal accounting controls over contributions received by mail:

— An outside agency may make test mailings of "contributions" that are subsequently traced into the records.
— An outside fund-raising service, having no access to cash receipts, may handle the mailing of all fund-raising literature and follow up on lack of adequate responses to campaigns.
— An organization may initiate confirmation procedures using previous contributor listings as the selection population.

DIRECT CONTACT SOLICITATIONS

If direct contact campaigns are conducted, the following are important controls:

— Appropriate supervision of the solicitors. This often is accomplished by a pyramid structure of area chairmen, division captains, neighborhood captains, and door-to-door solicitors, with each level reporting to the next higher level.
— Restriction of solicitation materials to authorized solicitors. This may involve a specific form of identification authorizing them to solicit contributions for the organization.
— Separation of physical control of cash from the accounting control over the contributions received. This separation should be achieved at the earliest possible point. For example, a door-to-door solicitor should submit a report to the neighborhood captain. The report should reconcile the contributions received (some of which may be

in the form of pledges) with the cash collected. The solicitor should also send a copy of the report directly to the organization's accounting department to establish accounting control and to permit later comparison with the amounts deposited.

— Minimization of the number of persons having access to cash and of the amount of cash in any one person's control. The cash collected should be deposited in a bank at the earliest practical time by a designated person (such as by the neighborhood captain).
— The use of fund-raising reports to check the results of each solicitation against street maps or other controls to ascertain that all areas and all solicitors have been accounted for.
— The use of prenumbered receipts, sponsor sheets, summary reports, etc. to ensure that all documents and related receipts are properly accounted for.
— Preparation of summaries of all fund-raising reports, reconciliation of all reports with the organization's records, and comparison of the recorded amounts with total bank deposits.
— Accounting for all sealed containers that are used to collect cash.

OTHER CONTROL PROCEDURES

Other internal accounting control procedures that may be appropriate for cash contributions include the following:

— Use of procedures similar to those for incoming mail to control the counting of the contents of sealed containers or of open plate collections. Containers, once collected, and open plate collections should be maintained under the joint control of two or more responsible persons until they are counted. The practice of using unattended, moveable, collection receptacles such as canisters or boxes is discouraged because incoming receipts are difficult to control and are subject to misdirection, misuse or theft.
— Establishment of separate accountabilities for donor-restricted gifts to appropriately classify and account for them and to monitor compliance with donor restrictions.
— Use of prenumbered contribution acknowledgment forms, when practicable.
— Maintenance of a record of gifts contingent on future events (such as bequests), which is reviewed periodically.
— Budgeting of contributions that can reasonably be estimated, and investigation of differences between actual contributions and such budgeted amounts or prior year amounts.
— Restrictive endorsement (for example: "for deposit only to the ac-

count of XYZ agency, account #65893 of First State Bank") of all checks received by the organization immediately upon receipt to prevent the deposit of such checks in unauthorized bank accounts.

— Publication of donors' names in a journal or program, and investigation of complaints from donors whose names were omitted, or the amount of whose gifts did not agree. The investigator should be a person who is independent of the contribution receiving and recording functions.

appendix 6

RATIO ANALYSIS*

To assist the users of *Standards* in analyzing an agency's financial statements, the following is a description of Ratio Analysis, an analytical tool used to assist boards and management of not-for-profit organizations and their contributing public in understanding organizations' financial statements.

APPLYING RATIO ANALYSIS

Ratios offer a capsulized view of key conditions affecting an agency's activities. The trend in these ratios reveals how an agency has changed over time. Since ratios and trends are often only indicators of a condition, it is precisely the intention of ratio analysis to help the interested party concentrate on those activities that warrant attention or are of concern. Ratio analysis also helps interested parties perform comparisons with other agencies that can be useful in identifying significant differences from the norms of comparison groups.

ASSESSMENT OF FINANCIAL CONDITION—BALANCE SHEET RATIOS

Ratio analysis helps users of financial statements to formulate answers to fundamental questions about the organization's financial status and performance, namely:

- Is the reporting organization clearly financially healthy or not as of the reporting date?
- Is the reporting organization financially better off or not at the end than it was at the beginning of the year reported on?

Readers of the organization's financial statements first should be concerned about its financial condition. There are two major ratios of financial condition which are called balance sheet ratios.

*This material is based largely on "Ratio Analysis in Voluntary Health and Welfare Organizations" (Peat, Marwick, Mitchell & Co., New York, NY 1982).

Ratio of Expendable Assets to Total Liabilities (Ratio No. 1)

This ratio indicates the relative liquidity of the organization. It is a fundamental indicator of financial strength. The numerator is composed of all assets, exclusive of land, buildings, and equipment and assets of endowment funds. The denominator is composed of all liabilities, including interfund borrowings, plant debt, and support and revenue designated for future periods. Ratio No.1 is derived from the concept that one of the most basic determinants of financial strength is the availability of sufficient cash, or assets that will convert to cash in the normal course of business, to meet all obligations as they come due. A ratio of 1:1 or greater indicates that, as of the balance sheet date, the organization had sufficient liquid assets to satisfy all related liabilities as well as plant debt.

For Voluntary Health and Welfare Service Affiliate, the ratio would be as follows: The numbers used in this ratio and the ratios to follow may be traced to Voluntary Health and Welfare Service Affiliate financial statements in Exhibit A, the Balance Sheet; Exhibit B, the Statement of Revenue and Expenses and Changes in Fund Balances; and Exhibit C, the Statement of Functional Expenses.

Calculation of Expendable Assets		Calulation of Ratio 1
Total Assets	$964,800	$\frac{\$595,200}{\$112,300} = 5.3:1$
Less: Fixed Assets	−174,800	
Less: Endowment Assets	−194,800	
Expendable Assets	$595,200	

This ratio indicates that Voluntary Health and Welfare Service Affiliate is financially viable because of the extensive expendable assets available to cover liabilities.

Ratio of Expendable Fund Balances to Total Expenses (Ratio No. 2)

This ratio describes the organization's ability to fund program and other expenses from expendable fund balances should no additional operating revenues be available. The numerator is composed of the following fund balances and deferred revenues at the end of the fiscal year, as reported on the balance sheet:

- Current funds—fund balances
- Current funds—contributions designated for future periods

The denominator is composed of all program services and supporting services expenses, excluding depreciation expense.

An appropriate ratio will depend on the size and nature of the organization and management's strategy for retaining fund balances.

For Voluntary Health and Welfare Service Affiliate, the ratio would be as follows:

Calculation of Expendable Fund Balances		Calculation of Expenses for Ratio	
Current fund balances:		Total Expenses	$720,600
Unrestricted	$485,100	Less: Depreciation	– 5,200
Restricted	6,400	Expenses for Ratio	$715,400
Support designated for future periods	18,000		
Expendable fund balances	$509,500		

Calculation of Ratio 2

$$\frac{\$509{,}500}{\$715{,}400} = .71{:}1$$

This ratio indicates that Voluntary Health and Welfare Service Affiliate has fund balances and deferred support sufficient to cover about two-thirds of its annual expenses.

EVALUATION OF FINANCIAL PERFORMANCE—CONTRIBUTION AND DEMAND RATIOS

Analysis of revenue by source, and expenses by function, can be prepared using ratios referred to as the "contribution and demand ratios." They address a third fundamental question that the analyst seeks to answer:

- Why have the organization's financial ratios behaved in the manner observed?

Contribution and demand ratios are most informative when reviewed as a trend over time.

Contribution Ratios

The contribution ratios that follow are derived from the main sources of revenue appearing on the voluntary health and welfare organization's Statement of Revenue and Expenses and Changes in Fund Balances. These contribution ratios are expressed as follows:

$$\frac{\text{Item of Revenue}}{\text{Total Expenses}}$$

These ratios indicate the contribution of the various sources of revenue to fund program services and other expenses. The numerator is the source of current funds *revenue* as presented on the Statement of Revenue and Expenses and Changes in Fund Balances. The denominator is defined as described for Ratio No. 2.

Two of the contribution ratios for a Voluntary Health and Welfare Service Affiliate are calculated as follows:

Ratio 3 and 4	Current Year
3. Contributions ($660,100 + 6,200)	
4. Allocated by federated fund-raising organizations	

Demand Ratios

Demand ratios are expressed as follows:

$$\frac{\text{Item of Expense}}{\text{Total Revenue}}$$

These ratios are especially useful in trend analyses in determining whether a particular category of expense is receiving a growing or dwindling share of the total revenue available. The numerator is the category of expense, exclusive of depreciation. The denominator is composed of current funds total revenue ($750,800 + 7,200 = $758,000).

Ratio 5 and 6	Current Year
5. Program Services—Program D ($257,800 – 2,900)	$\frac{\$254,900}{\$758,000} = 34\%$
6. Supporting Services—Management and General ($57,400 – 600)	$\frac{\$\ 56,800}{\$758,000} = 7\%$

FUND-RAISING RATIOS

Many contributors and government regulators compute ratios of fund-raising costs to funds raised, and there is ongoing discussion of appropriate ratios and comparisons of organizations. There are numerous factors that make calculation and comparison of such ratios misleading. Those factors include:

- *Federated Fund-Raising Costs Omitted*—Many agencies, in addition to support from the public that they obtain directly, receive public support indirectly through federated and other fund-raising organizations whose fund-raising costs are not included in the reporting agency's financial statements.
- *Differing Time Periods for Revenue and Expenses*—Bequests or government grants, that may be unsolicited or received years after they were solicited, may preclude any meaningful matching of support and revenue with fund-raising costs.
- *Use of Volunteers*—Many agencies receive significant assistance from volunteers in their fund-raising efforts. The assistance may vary in size and quality from agency to agency and may or may not be includable in contributions and fund-raising costs.
- *Forms of Solicitation*—Some agencies have higher fund-raising costs because the fund-raising methods available to them are inherently more costly—e.g., direct mail vs. certain forms of personal solicitation.

Accordingly, factors other than the support and fund-raising costs, as they appear in the annual financial statements, must be considered whenever fund-raising ratios are calculated.

appendix 7

REPORTING OF SERVICE EFFORTS AND ACCOMPLISHMENTS

As previously noted, Concepts Statement No. 4 suggests that service efforts and accomplishments information is useful in assessing an organization's performance. Such information is useful because accomplishments of not-for-profit organizations generally cannot be measured solely by traditional financial indicators, and because resource providers who are not beneficiaries or recipients of an organization's services often do not have direct knowledge about an organization's outputs.

Service efforts generally refer to inputs—money, personnel, and materials—which comprise the costs of providing programs and services. Most organizations present service efforts information in their financial statements through functional expense reporting. Service accomplishments generally refers to outputs—goods or services produced and program results. Techniques for reporting this information are generally less developed than those for service efforts, and, for that reason, FASB Concepts Statement No. 4 uses the qualifying language "*ideally* [emphasis added] financial reporting also should provide information about the service accomplishments of a nonbusiness organization."

In 1980, the FASB published the results of a study commissioned by the Board to review not-for-profit organizations' financial reports and to record and classify instances in which the organizations reported their performance using service efforts and accomplishments information. The study concluded that most service efforts and accomplishments reporting was done in reports other than general purpose external financial reports. In addition, information about efforts was more prevalent than information about accomplishments. Information about results was noted less frequently, and the study suggested that additional research in the area should be encouraged. Currently, the Governmental Accounting Standards Board is studying the topic.

Until additional research on the topic is completed, no standards on reporting service accomplishments will be issued. Nevertheless, agencies are encouraged to experiment with presenting this information with the objective of improving the communication of their achievements to constituencies.

appendix 8

ACCOUNTING FOR JOINT COSTS OF INFORMATIONAL MATERIALS AND ACTIVITIES THAT INCLUDE A FUND-RAISING APPEAL

As discussed in Chapter V, in certain circumstances, voluntary health and welfare organizations should allocate the joint costs of informational materials and activities that include a fund-raising appeal between the fund-raising function and the appropriate program or management and general function. While Statement of Position 87-2 (SOP) issued by the American Institute of Certified Public Accountants provides the conceptual base needed to identify circumstances in which such allocation is appropriate, significant practical questions regarding the interpretation of the SOP and the techniques for cost allocation must be resolved by each individual agency.

This appendix has been prepared to provide some insights into these issues. While many questions undoubtedly will continue to plague those who must deal with this matter, it is anticipated that consensus will develop over time and that the next edition of *Standards* will include the benefit of that experience. In the meantime, it is hoped that the guidance offered in the following discussion will contribute to the achievement of the goal that well-intentioned individuals arrive at reasonably the same conclusions when faced with the same facts. This will help to retain and enhance the credibility of the financial reports presented to the contributing public by voluntary health and welfare agencies.

BONA FIDE PROGRAM OR MANAGEMENT AND GENERAL FUNCTION

All joint costs should be charged to fund raising unless it can be demonstrated that a bona fide program or management and general function has been conducted in conjunction with an appeal for funds. Whether a bona fide management and general function has been conducted in connection with an appeal is often clear. For example, preparation and distribution of an annual report is a management and general function, since it represents the fulfillment of the stewardship responsibility to account to donors on the use of the resources made available to the agency. Accordingly, if an appeal for funds is made at the same time that the annual report is distributed to prior contributors, a bona fide management and general function will have been carried out in the joint activity.

The determination of the degree to which a bona fide program activity has been conducted in connection with the appeal, however, is often less clear. In assessing this issue, the organization must focus on its basic mission to determine whether that mission includes purposes which are accomplished by the dissemination of information. For many not-for-profit organizations, this review will result in a conclusion that a bona fide information program activity does not exist. Mere communication of the nature of the cause and of the programs which the organization conducts to deal with it, does not justify a determination that a bona fide program has been conducted. Rather, it must be clear that in order to accomplish a portion of its basic reason for being, the agency must disseminate information.

Many voluntary health agencies have as a basic mission the communication of health information of benefit to the recipient. This information is problem-oriented rather than agency-oriented and is designed to motivate action on the part of the recipient. In these circumstances, it may clearly be concluded that the agency is conducting a bona fide program which contributes directly to the accomplishment of its basic mission.

DEMONSTRATING THAT PROGRAM IS BONA FIDE

To justify allocation of joint costs, the Statement of Position requires that verifiable indications of the reasons for conducting the program portion of the activity be present. These indications presumably will permit verification by the agency's independent auditors, state regulators or others of the propriety of the conclusion that costs should be allocated. These indications include:

1. *Content of the non-fundraising portion of the activity*. The substance of the content and the degree to which it may be concluded that the dissemination of the information is cost justified in the accomplishment of mission is critical. In other words, it must be determinable that the content of the non-fundraising element is significant in its own right and that its inclusion in the joint activity is a cost-effective way to accomplish a portion of the agency's program objectives.
2. *Audience targeted*. The nature of the audience to which the joint effort is directed is also significant in assessing the legitimacy of the program element. For example, selection of only known wealthy individuals or prior large givers for the audience to which the activity is directed may lead to a conclusion that while the agency may otherwise conduct bona fide infor-

mational programs, a bona fide program activity was not conducted in connection with this appeal. In some circumstances, however, dissemination of program information to wealthy individuals may directly contribute to accomplishment of mission if those individuals are able to take actions (other than contributing) which those less affluent might not be able to take.

It is also important in addressing the issue of targeted audience to recognize that the mere fact that an agency communicates with prior givers does not automatically lead to a conclusion that the program element of the activity is not bona fide. In fact, prior givers have, by virtue of those gifts, demonstrated an interest in the cause for which the agency exists. Accordingly, where the accomplishment of the programs for which the organization exists legitimately includes dissemination of information which will result in action by the recipient, communication with prior donors often is an effective way to fulfill those programs.

3. *Action requested.* As indicated, the non-fundraising information must be problem-oriented and designed to motivate the audience to action in order for the program element to be bona fide. This action may range from personal changes in health habits to participation in efforts to modify legislation. It must, however, be clear that the information is not merely a statement of the purposes for which the agency seeks support.
4. *Other corroborating evidence.* Written instructions to media consultants, board minutes, narrative budget data and similar documentation of the reasons for the program element of the activity should be retained to assist in providing verifiable indications that the program element is bona fide. For example, it would be expected that medical and other health professionals, rather than fund-raising consultants, would create literature or other information pieces dealing with health agency programs. Documentation of annual program objectives, specific program activities to accomplish those objectives and evidence of professional medical clearance of health-related public messages would be normal types of corroborating evidence to support a conclusion regarding the bona fides of a public health education program. Alternatively, even though the program objective might be bona fide, the accomplishment of that objective in a joint activity might be questioned. For example, in circumstances where paid solicitors are used to conduct the activity, particularly if compensation is based upon funds raised, the legitimacy of the program element might be suspect.

COST ALLOCATION

In applying these concepts to the day-to-day activities of a voluntary health or welfare agency, all of the circumstances surrounding the joint activity must be considered together and a conclusion must be reached that is supported by the facts. Once it has been determined that a bona fide joint program or management and general function has been conducted together with a fund-raising appeal, costs should be allocated equitably to the respective functions.

While concern has been expressed about the need for more specific guidance regarding techniques for allocating costs, accountants understand that the application of normal cost accounting techniques will result in allocations that will fairly reflect the purposes for which the activity was conducted. Voluntary health and welfare organizations have for many years maintained accounting systems to allocate the costs of salaries, rent, telephone and other operating expenses to the program, fund raising or management and general functions for which the costs were incurred. In some cases, this requires time reports, estimates of space usage and other cost accounting techniques to be employed (see Appendix 1 for a discussion of this topic).

The allocation of joint costs should be based essentially upon the degree to which the cost element was incurred for fund raising or for other function purposes. It is important to understand that the issue of allocation of joint costs deals solely with the allocation of that pool of expenses which are ***not*** directly identifiable with fund raising or another function. Those which are identified with a specific function should be charged to that function directly in the normal accounting process.

DISCLOSURE

As illustrated in Chapter V, the notes to the financial statements should disclose that joint costs have been allocated whenever material in amount, including the amount of the total pool of joint costs and the amount allocated to fund raising, management and general or specific program functions.

EXAMPLES

The following examples have been developed to assist agencies in dealing with the issues encountered in typical circumstances. It is again emphasized, however, that each agency and each activity is unique and that all circumstances must be evaluated on an overall basis in preparing financial statements which fairly reflect an agency's use of resources.

Coordinated Mail Program

With the advent of computerized techniques for mass mailings and the increasing sophistication of direct mail fund raising, many agencies have developed coordinated mail programs to accomplish a portion of their program objectives, recruit volunteers and raise funds to support future programs. While the problems associated with joint costs of informational materials and activities which include a fund-raising appeal apply to other types of fund raising, the relative amount of joint costs involved in direct mail programs causes this to be the area of greater concern for most agencies.

Joint costs of direct mail activities include the postage, envelopes and computer costs, but may also include the cost of the message. To help substantiate the validity of the program element of the activity, it is helpful if the program message is printed on a separate piece or in a separate box or panel from the fund-raising appeal. While not always possible, this permits use of the respective pieces in other than direct mail activities while avoiding the difficulty of attempting to attribute program or fund-raising purposes to the individual lines of a joint message. In assessing whether a bona fide program activity has been conducted, the lack of a separate program piece or separate box or panel developed by the related program staff may contribute to a conclusion that there is a lack of verifiable evidence of the existence of substantive programs.

Mail Example 1

An organization maintains a list of its prior contributors to whom it sends donor renewal mailings which include program messages on a separate piece. When prior donors have not given for a number of years, they are deleted from the list.

Since the organization selects individuals to be added to or deleted from the list based on their presumed ability to provide financial support, it might be concluded that all joint costs should be charged to fund raising. (The direct costs of the separate program piece would be charged to programs in any event.) However, if verifiable indications exist that a bona fide program activity was conducted, this presumption might be overcome. For example, if the minutes of the program committee reflected a discussion of the most cost-effective techniques available to reach people with an interest in the agency's cause and the separate program message requesting action by the recipient which would contribute to the accomplishment of the agency's basic mission was prepared by medical staff, allocation of the joint costs might be justified.

Mail Example 2

An organization conducts an annual fund-raising mailing which includes a flyer telling what to do about an environmental problem. Mailing labels in selected ZIP Code areas are purchased from a list supplier. The ZIP Codes are selected based upon income levels using census data. The higher income ZIP Codes are included. The lower income ZIP Codes are excluded.

Because the audience selection is based upon its presumed ability to provide financial support, an initial reaction might be that all joint costs should be charged to fund raising. (Again, the direct costs of a separate program piece would be charged to program in any event.) However, it would be necessary to review the verifiable indications of bona fide program activity associated with the content of the program message, the actions requested and other corroborating evidence as well as the targeted audience before a conclusion could be reached. In this case, it might be determined that the action requested involved organizing community efforts to modify legislation regarding the environmental problems, a result that might reasonably be expected to be more readily accomplished in the specific circumstances of this agency by marshalling the efforts of residents of more affluent communities.

Mail Example 3

An organization's mailing list broker recommends lists to be tested for fund-raising results. A small percentage of the names is randomly selected from each list for testing. Each letter contains bona fide program and fund-raising messages. The number and amount of contributions received through each test mailing provides the basis for projecting fund-raising results. Only if these fund-raising projections are satisfactory are additional names rented or exchanged for continuation mailings.

Since the audience selections are based on the presumption that the mailings will provide financial support, regardless of the audiences' need for or interest in the program messages, only the direct costs clearly identifiable with the program messages are charged to program. All joint costs of the test mailings should be charged to the fund-raising function.

Mail Example 4

A society for senior citizens mails a brochure on the importance of exercise in later years to residents over the age of 58 in three ZIP Codes. The last two pages of the four-page brochure include a perforated contribution remittance form on which the society explains its program and makes an appeal for funds. The content of the first two pages of the brochure is primarily educational (about exercise) and explains how seniors can undertake a self-supervised exercise program and urges them to do so.

The reasons for distributing the leaflet are to educate this age group about the need to exercise and to raise funds for the society. This is documented in a letter to the public relations firm that developed the piece and is supported by the approval of a medical advisory board to the exercise program. The audience is selected based on age, without regard to ability to contribute. The society considered that almost all of the recipients would benefit personally from the information about exercise and that the recipients were not selected on their ability to contribute. In this case, joint costs should be allocated to both program and fund-raising functions.

Residential Campaign

Residential fund-raising campaigns in which volunteers canvass their neighborhoods for support have also been used by many organizations as a cost-effective way to disseminate legitimate program messages. However, changes in our society have made these campaigns less effective from a fund-raising standpoint in recent years due to such factors as two-career families, an increasingly mobile population and concerns about street crime. Nevertheless, even though these campaigns often raise less than in prior years, certain agencies have continued them because of the importance of the program aspects of the effort. In these circumstances, it may sometimes be concluded that the fund-raising objectives are incidental to the program objectives and that joint costs should be allocated to the program function. Joint costs in residential appeals typically include the cost of volunteer recruitment and solicitor kits.

An issue in volunteer recruitment often involves the allocation of related telephone costs. Typically, volunteers or paid recruiters use the phones to contact other residents in the community to solicit their participation in the residential drive. Often, the individuals placing the calls will read a message to the person answering the phone which imparts a program message and requests his or her involvement as a volunteer. If a review of the verifiable indications of a bona fide program element in the *drive* confirms its legitimacy, a basis exists for allocation of the telephone recruitment costs, as well as the other joint costs of the drive itself. While an approach might be to allocate costs of the telephones and paid recruiters based on the percentage that the program message which is read over the phone bears to the total message, it is doubtful that many cases exist in which this approach is supportable. It is unlikely that agencies would create programs of public education, for example, which would be deemed to be sufficiently effective by simply reading a brief message over the telephone to justify the costs involved. However, these costs might properly be allocable based upon the mix of bona fide programs and fund-raising activities which the recruited volunteers are asked to perform during the residential drive since the recruitment of volunteers is an essential element of a successful drive.

Some agencies directly solicit contributions over the phone, often combining a program message with the appeal. For similar reasons of lack of substance and cost effectiveness regarding the program aspect of this activity, all joint costs would normally be charged to fund raising.

Residential Example 1

An environmental group conducts a door-to-door canvass of a community which is affected by recent adverse environmental conditions. The canvassers inform the residents about the environmental problems; seek signatures on a petition; recommend other actions residents could take to help eliminate the problems; and ask for donations. The ability of the residents of this community to provide financial support is not a basis for selection, none of the residents are included because of their presumed ability to provide support or excluded because of their lack thereof, and all neighborhoods are covered.

Since the audience is selected based on their presumed need for, or interest in the program messages without regard to their ability to provide financial support, only the direct costs clearly identifiable with including a request for funds during the canvass are charged to fund-raising expense. All joint costs are charged to the program function since the fund raising is incidental to the activity in these circumstances.

Residential Example 2

An agency conducts a door-to-door solicitation campaign for a camp program for disadvantaged youth. In the campaign, volunteers visit homes in middle class neighborhoods with canisters. The volunteers explain the camp's programs, including why the disadvantaged children benefit from the program, and distribute leaflets to the residents regardless of whether they contribute to the camp. The leaflets describe the camp, its activities, who can attend, and the benefits to attendees. Requests for contributions are *not* included in the leaflets.

In evaluating how the cost of this campaign should be treated, the following should be considered:

- The canisters were used solely to collect contributions;
- The leaflets described the camp, but did not encourage any action from the reader;
- The volunteers visited residents of middle class neighborhoods that management expected would not need the camp's programs but would be in a position to contribute.

In this case, all costs of this campaign should be charged to fund-raising expense.

If the same scenario was moved to a disadvantaged neighborhood, and residents were also given a phone number to call or an address to write to for more information, the conclusion would be different. In those circumstances, only the cost of the canisters would be charged to fund raising since the fund raising would be incidental to the program purpose. The information about the program and how to take advantage of it would be charged to program expense.

Telethon

Television and radio provide significant opportunities for voluntary health and welfare organizations to reach the public with program messages while soliciting funds. Allocation of joint costs in these instances requires a review of the verifiable indications of the bona fide nature of the program element. Once it has been concluded that the agency does, in fact, accomplish an element of its basic mission by communicating with the public, a basis for allocation of joint costs may be developed by review of the content of the telethon. This may be done by examining the show log which should reflect the on-air time and content of each segment of the show. Joint costs of telethons may include such elements as amounts of air time, production and broadcasting costs. Costs of "800" numbers for pledge purposes should be charged to fund raising.

Telethon Example

An organization conducts an annual national telethon to raise funds and to reach the American public with life-saving educational messages. The broadcast includes segments on personal health care and other segments describing the organization's services. The organization broadcasts the telethon to the entire country and not just to areas selected on the basis of giving potential or prior fund-raising results.

Since the audience selection is random and not based either on the presumption that the audiences selected will provide financial support or on the audiences' need for or interest in the program messages, the direct costs clearly identifiable with the personal health care messages should be charged to the program function. The costs of the service description messages which inform the audience about the organization and the related appeal for funds should be charged to fund raising. Joint costs such as TV time, overall planning, and production should be allocated between program and fund raising based upon the relative amounts of time each was on the air.

• • • • •

Allocation of costs by voluntary health and welfare organizations is required to permit the readers of financial statements to understand the purposes for which funds were expended (programs, fund raising or management and general) and not solely the nature of costs (salaries, rent, telephone, etc.). This requires the exercise of judgment and an understanding of the accounting definitions of program, fund raising and management and general. While inherently subjective, this process provides more meaningful information if done with care and integrity. Agencies are urged to carefully plan the techniques which will be employed to document the basis on which allocations are made and to assure that the result is a fair reflection of the actual activities which have taken place.

INDEX

G

H

I

J

L

M

N

Q

R

S

T

U

V

W